RAND Health

Improving Childhood Asthma Outcomes in the United States

A Blueprint for Policy Action

Marielena Lara • Will Nicholas • Sally Morton • Mary E. Vaiana
Barbara Genovese • Gary Rachelefsky

with a National Expert Committee Co-Chaired by
Stephen Redd and Kevin Weiss

Supported by the Robert Wood Johnson Foundation

RAND

The research described in this report was sponsored by the Robert Wood Johnson Foundation.

Library of Congress Cataloging-in-Publication Data

Improving childhood asthma outcomes in the United States / Marielena Lara ...
[et. al.].
p. cm.
"MR-1330."
Includes bibliographical references.
ISBN 0-8330-2997-5
1. Asthma in children—Government policy—United States. I. Lara, Marielena.

RJ436.A8 I475 2001
362.1'9892238'00973—dc21

2001019562

Published 2001 by RAND
1700 Main Street, P.O. Box 2138, Santa Monica, CA 90407-2138
1200 South Hayes Street, Arlington, VA 22202-5050
201 North Craig Street, Suite 102, Pittsburgh, PA 15213-1516
RAND URL: http://www.rand.org/
To order RAND documents or to obtain additional information, contact Distribution Services: Telephone: (310) 451-7002;
Fax: (310) 451-6915; Internet: order@rand.org

PREFACE

An estimated 5 million U.S. children have asthma. Too many of these children are unnecessarily impaired. Much of the money spent on asthma is for high-cost health care services to treat acute periods of illness. Many asthma attacks could be avoided—and much suffering prevented and many medical costs saved—if more children received good-quality, ongoing asthma care and if the 11 policy recommendations presented in this report were implemented in a coordinated fashion.

This report is dedicated to children with asthma and their caregivers. It summarizes the findings of an effort funded by the Robert Wood Johnson Foundation, to

- Identify a range of policy actions in both the public and private sectors that could improve childhood asthma outcomes nationwide
- Select a subset of policies to create a blueprint for national policy in this area
- Outline alternatives to implement these policies that build on prior efforts.

To conduct this work, RAND Health engaged an interdisciplinary panel of nationally recognized leaders in childhood asthma in a structured group process to identify the policy recommendations proposed in this report. This process, which included a face-to-face expert committee meeting, led to the development of a comprehensive policy framework that maps the identified strategies to one overall policy objective: to promote the development and maintenance of *asthma-friendly communities*—communities in which children with asthma are swiftly diagnosed, receive appropriate and ongoing treatment, and are not exposed to environmental factors that exacerbate their condition.

The 11 policy recommendations presented in this report are a national call to action. The recommendations span public and private interests and involve the integration of public health activities across local, state, and federal levels.

The intent of the blueprint is to provide inspiration for innovative ways to strengthen the collaboration and communication among national and local community leaders and programs, and to successfully translate these national policies into local community practices.

This effort is part of the Robert Wood Johnson Foundation's Pediatric Asthma Initiative. The purpose of this initiative is to address current gaps in national childhood asthma care through clinical and nonclinical approaches to improve the management of childhood asthma. It is the first national initiative that simultaneously addresses treatment, policy, and financing issues for children with asthma at the patient, provider, and institutional levels.

The report is based on research conducted under the auspices of RAND Health. RAND Health furthers RAND's mission of helping improve policy and decisionmaking through research and analysis, by working to improve health care systems and advance understanding of how the organization and financing of care affect costs, quality, and access.

NATIONAL EXPERT COMMITTEE MEMBERS AND RAND HEALTH STAFF

NATIONAL EXPERT COMMITTEE MEMBERS

Stephen Redd
Committee Co-Chair
Chief, Air Pollution and Respiratory
Health Branch
Centers for Disease Control and Prevention

Noreen Clark
Dean, Marshall H. Becker
Professor of Public Health
University of Michigan

Nicole Lurie
(Formerly) Principal Deputy
Assistant Secretary for Health
Department of Health and
Human Services

Thomas Platts-Mills
Director, Asthma and Allergic
Diseases Center
University of Virginia

Kevin Weiss
Committee Co-Chair
Director, Center for Healthcare
Studies
Northwestern Medical School

Sara Rosenbaum
Director, Center for Health
Services Research and Policy
The George Washington
University School of Public
Health and Health Services

Vernon Smith
Principal
Health Management Associates

Lani Wheeler
Pediatric and School Health
Consultant
Anne Arundel County
Department of Health
Maryland

RAND HEALTH STAFF

Marielena Lara
Principal Investigator

Gary Rachelefsky
Co-Principal Investigator
Allergy Research Foundation

Sally Morton
Head, Statistics Group

Mary E. Vaiana
Communications Director

Will Nicholas
Associate Policy Analyst

Marian Branch
Editor

Barbara Genovese
Project Manager

Carolyn Rogers and
Alaida Rodríguez
Administrative Assistants

LIST OF EXTERNAL REVIEWERS

Agency for Healthcare Research and Quality
Denise M. Dougherty, Ph.D.
Senior Advisor, Child Health

American Academy of Allergy, Asthma & Immunology
Gail G. Shapiro, M.D.
President-Elect

American Academy of Family Physicians
Herbert F. Young, M.D., M.A.
Director, Scientific Activities Division
Barbara P. Yawn, M.D., M.Sc.
Director of Research, Olmsted Medical Center

American Academy of Pediatrics
Robert A. Wood, M.D.
Section on Allergy and Immunology Executive Committee
Department of Pediatrics, School of Medicine
The Johns Hopkins Hospital

American Academy of Physician Assistants
Gabriel Ortiz, M.P.A.S., P.A.

American Association of Health Plans
Peter Fitzgerald, M.Sc.
Director, Quality Management and Health Services Research

American College of Allergy, Asthma & Immunology
Emil J. Bardana, Jr., M.D.
President
William Storms, M.D.
Asthma and Allergy Associates, Colorado Springs, CO

American College of Emergency Physicians

American Lung Association
Fran DuMelle
Executive Vice President

American Pharmaceutical Foundation
William M. Ellis, R.Ph., M.S.
Executive Director

American Public Health Association
Larry K. Olsen, Dr.P.H., CHES
Chair, School Health Education and Services Section

American Public Human Services Association
Lee Partridge
Director of the Health Policy Unit
Erin Nagy
Health Policy Analyst

American Thoracic Society
William J. Martin, II, M.D.
President

Asthma & Allergy Foundation of America
Mary Worstell, M.P.H.
Executive Director

Asthma and Allergy Network/Mothers of Asthmatics
Nancy Sander
President

Environmental Protection Agency
Mary T. Smith
Director, Indoor Environments Division

Health Care Financing Administration

Timothy M. Westmoreland
Director, Center for Medicaid and State Operations

M. Beth Benedict, R.N., Dr.P.H., J.D.
Social Science Research Analyst
Office of Strategic Planning

Beverly Koops, M.D.
Medical Director, Health Care Financing
Texas Department of Health

Health Resources and Services Administration

Peter C. van Dyck, M.D., M.P.H.
Associate Administrator
Maternal and Child Health Bureau

National Committee for Quality Assurance

L. Gregory Pawlson, M.D., M.P.H.
Executive Vice President

National Heart, Lung, and Blood Institute

Claude Lenfant, M.D.
Director and Chair of the National Asthma
Education and Prevention Committee

Virginia Taggart, M.P.H.
Division of Lung Diseases

Diana Schmidt
Coordinator, National Asthma Education and Prevention Committee

Robinson Fulwood, Ph.D., M.S.P.H.
Senior Manager, Office of Prevention, Education, and Control

National Institute of Allergy and Infectious Diseases

Anthony S. Fauci, M.D.
Director

National Institute of Child Health and Human Development

Duane Alexander, M.D.
Director

National Institute of Environmental Health Sciences
Kenneth Olden, Ph.D.
Director

Pacific Business Group on Health
Cheryl Damberg, Ph.D.
Director of Research and Quality

Society for Academic Emergency Medicine
Brian J. Zink, M.D.
President
Jill Baren, M.D., FAAP
Chair, Pediatric Interest Group
Carlos Camargo, M.D., Dr.P.H.
Assistant Professor of Medicine
Harvard Medical School

University of California, Los Angeles; and RAND Health
Arleen Leibowitz, Ph.D.
Chair, Department of Policy Studies

U.S. Department of Education
Debra Price-Ellingstad, Ed.D.
Education Program Specialist
Office of Special Education Programs

U.S. Department of Housing and Urban Development
Warren Friedman, Ph.D., CIH

CONTENTS

IMPROVING CHILDHOOD ASTHMA OUTCOMES IN THE UNITED STATES: A BLUEPRINT FOR POLICY ACTION

Almost everyone knows a child with asthma. Although asthma is a treatable disease, too many children with asthma suffer unnecessarily. Some even die. Yet children whose asthma is properly controlled can lead fully active lives, with minimal symptoms.

The number of persons with asthma in the United States has doubled in the past 15 years. Children are the most affected: An estimated 5 million children under 15 years old have this disease. The cases of asthma in children under 5 years old increased more than 160 percent between 1980 and 1994. For children ages 5 to 14, the increase was 74 percent. Asthma is more common among children who are poor, African American, or Puerto Rican.

The costs and consequences of childhood asthma

The disease has serious economic consequences. Asthma cost an estimated $10.7 billion in 1994—more than half of it for direct medical expenses, the rest for indirect costs associated with school and work days lost, as well as with premature mortality. A significant portion of the medical expenses was for tertiary care, such as hospitalizations and emergency room visits.

Medical care for asthma has improved significantly. Effective primary care can help children with asthma to lead fully functional lives and prevent costly hospitalizations.

Yet the human and financial costs of childhood asthma continue to grow.

Why? One major reason is that we still do not know enough about the causes of asthma and its progression. We know that a variety of risk factors, including a genetic predisposition, environmental exposure, poverty, and inadequate heath care services, play a role in asthma—but we do not know their precise effects or how they interact with each other. Another major reason is that the complexity of this public health problem points toward solutions involving many different organizations and sectors of U.S. society.

Childhood asthma is a national public health problem that challenges not only the entire health system but also school systems and the many public and private organizations that track the effects of this illness, provide education and other community-based programs, and fund research into the causes of asthma. Improving care for childhood asthma will require better coordination of ongoing national efforts, as well as a significant commitment of national resources. Equally important is the commitment of individual state and local organizations and individual communities nationwide. Success will depend on integrating local, state, and national efforts.

Our purpose and approach

In October 1999, the Robert Wood Johnson Foundation funded RAND Health to outline future directions for childhood asthma policy in the United States. The purposes of this effort, conducted as part of a broader Pediatric Asthma Initiative sponsored by the Foundation, were to

- Identify a range of policy actions in both the public and private sectors that could improve childhood asthma outcomes nationwide.
- Select a subset of policies to create a blueprint for national policy in this area.
- Outline alternatives to implement these policies that build on prior efforts.

RAND Health engaged an interdisciplinary panel of nationally recognized leaders in childhood asthma, the National Expert Committee, in a structured group process. The panel identified 11 policy recommendations that form a comprehensive framework for achieving one broad policy objective: to promote the development and maintenance of *asthma-friendly* communities.

Policy objective: **asthma-friendly** *communities nationwide*

In an *asthma-friendly community,* children with asthma are quickly diagnosed and receive appropriate and ongoing treatment; health care, school, and social agencies are prepared to meet the needs of children with asthma and their families; and children are safe from physical and social environmental risks that exacerbate asthma.

Policy goals

The RAND panel also identified six policy goals to meet its objective of promoting *asthma-friendly* communities:

- **Improve access to and quality of asthma health care services.**
- **Improve asthma awareness among affected individuals and the general public.**
- **Ensure *asthma-friendly* schools.**
- **Promote *asthma-safe* home environments.**
- **Encourage innovation in asthma prevention and management**
- **Reduce socioeconomic disparities in childhood asthma outcomes.**

Translating goals into 11 policy recommendations

The panel's policy recommendations for meeting these goals span public and private interests and call for the integration of public health activities across local, state, and federal levels. The 11 recommendations fall into two broad areas, and are described below:

- **Improving health care delivery and financing**

Recommendations in this area are designed to

- — Promote quality of care for key childhood asthma care services (Recommendations 1, 2, and 3).
- — Increase access to these services by expanding insurance coverage, improving benefits design, and educating health care purchasers (Recommendations 4, 5, and 6).

- **Strengthening the public health infrastructure**

These recommendations are directed at the government agencies responsible for administering and financing public health functions that support and supplement the health care delivery system. They are designed to

- — Publicly fund asthma-related community and health services that fall outside the health insurance system (Recommendations 7 and 8).
- — Increase public awareness and knowledge of asthma (Recommendation 9).
- — Improve surveillance and prevention research efforts (Recommendations 10 and 11).

RECOMMENDATIONS FOR IMPROVING HEALTH CARE DELIVERY AND FINANCING

1. Develop and implement primary care performance measures for childhood asthma care

Although evidence-based guidelines are available for childhood asthma, there is a substantial gap between accepted best practices for asthma care and the care delivered in the primary care setting. The Committee recommends that health care regulators, insurers, and health care delivery organizations implement the use of primary-care performance measures for childhood asthma. To encourage adherence to guidelines health care organizations would use provider-education strategies of proven effectiveness and offer financial incentives. In the absence of universal access to primary care, special efforts to improve coordination between primary and emergency care are necessary.

Implementation Options. The National Asthma Education and Prevention Program (NAEPP) would play a key role in coordinating the dissemination of childhood asthma care guidelines to insurers, managed care organizations, and state agencies for Medicaid and for the State Children's Health Insurance Program. Quality monitoring organizations such as the National Committee for Quality Assurance (NCQA) would work with the NAEPP, professional organizations, and parent organizations to incorporate asthma-care performance measures into NCQA's HEDIS (Health Plan Employer Data and Information Set) performance measurement system or into alternative quality measurement systems. These efforts could draw on previous successful models for guideline implementation and performance measurement for diabetes and cancer.

Funding Options. Federal funding would support NAEPP's expanded role in maintaining up-to-date guidelines. The NAEPP could also solicit funding from private sources to supplement these activities, as was done for the publication of the original guidelines. Funding for the development of performance measures could be sought from the pharmaceutical industry, Health Care Financing Administration, and NCQA. Other funding for updating and disseminating quality performance measures would continue to come from the health care and health insurance organizations that now perform these tasks.

2. Teach all children with persistent asthma and their families a specific set of self-management skills

Educating patients about their disease can improve their ability to manage the disease and prevent complications that lead to hospitalizations and emergency department visits. The Committee recommends that the National Asthma Education and Prevention Program (NAEPP) use its current recommendations for asthma self-management education to develop and disseminate a specific set of patient-education performance measures to be used for quality monitoring; that education materials meet patients' language and literacy requirements; and that health care purchasers and providers encourage asthma education for all children with persistent asthma.

Implementation Options. The NAEPP, in collaboration with appropriate professional organizations, would take the lead in establishing performance measures for the content of asthma education and self-management programs and in disseminating these measures. The National Committee for Quality Assurance and other quality monitoring organizations would work with the NAEPP to incorporate these measures into NCQA's HEDIS performance measurement system or into alternative quality monitoring systems. Professional and lay organizations would be involved in the development of educational materials for patients and their families and would work closely with their local affiliates to implement asthma patient education at the local facility level.

Funding Options. Efforts to establish performance measures would be funded by the federal government and private philanthropic organizations. Collaborative funding from the pharmaceutical industry could also be sought. Funding for the provision of asthma self-management education to patients would be covered by public and private insurers as allowed by federal and state laws (see Recommendations 5–6). For children without health insurance, these services would be covered through the public health infrastructure (see Recommendation 7).

3. Provide case-management to high-risk children

Asthma case-management is a comprehensive set of services, provided by teams of medical professionals and social work staff, that includes intensive tracking, coordinated care, and follow-up. Case-management increases the effectiveness of patient education and reduces morbidity and use of emergency services among inner-city children with asthma. Because case-management services are expensive, it makes sense to focus them on high-risk children.

The Committee recommends that the National Asthma Education and Prevention Program (NAEPP) develop evidence-based performance measures for case-management, and that health care purchasers and providers encourage their use among all high-risk children with asthma.

Implementation Options. The NAEPP and the Agency for Healthcare Research and Quality Asthma Evidence-based Practice Center would take the lead in synthesizing existing research on asthma case-management. Professional organizations would disseminate these guidelines to providers, targeting those in high-risk areas. The American Association of Health Plans and managed care organizations could encourage their health plans to provide case-management services. State Medicaid and State Children's Health Insurance Program programs could ensure that all contracting plans have the capacity to provide case-management services to high-risk areas. The Health Resources and Services Administration could ensure the same for federally funded community health centers.

Funding Options. Funding for updating and disseminating quality performance measures for case-management would continue to come from the organizations that now perform these tasks. The pharmaceutical industry could also provide collaborative funding. Case-management services would be funded through public and private health insurers (see Recommendation 5) and the public health infrastructure (see Recommendation 7).

4. Extend continuous health insurance coverage to all uninsured children

All children need health insurance, and continuous insurance coverage is critical for improving the health of children with asthma. Existing insurance mechanisms can go a long way toward achieving the goal of insuring all children. In concert, the current Medicaid and State Children's Health Insurance Program (SCHIP) programs have the potential to ensure that virtually all children have access to health insurance coverage, regardless of family income. But even with vigorous state efforts, two groups of children would remain at risk of being uninsured: children of working parents who do not qualify for public insurance but do not have insurance from their employers, and children who are not citizens.

The committee recommends that Congress extend continuous health insurance coverage to all uninsured children; that states make maximum use of Medicaid and SCHIP; and that federal and state policies create incentives for employers to offer affordable coverage to all workers with children, and extend coverage to all children residing in the United States, regardless of legal status.

Implementation Options. Asthma-related organizations would develop collaborations to educate state governments about the importance of improving Medicaid and SCHIP coverage, as well as the importance of new laws that encourage employers to furnish affordable coverage. They would also educate health insurance and small-business organizations about the importance of providing affordable coverage to workers. Potential beneficiaries would be made aware of expanded eligibility and coverage.

Funding Options. Federal and state governments would need to appropriate additional funds to expand eligibility and coverage for public insurance. Through direct appropriation or tax incentives, Congress could encourage employers to offer family coverage at subsidized rates. Congress would also have to pass legislation to make noncitizen children who meet program requirements eligible for full coverage under Medicaid and SCHIP.

5. Develop model benefit packages for essential childhood asthma services

Children with asthma must have insurance benefit packages that reflect appropriate performance standards of childhood asthma care. But certain services essential for proper treatment of these children may not be routinely covered by private health insurance plans and may not be covered under state SCHIP plans maintained separately from Medicaid.

The Committee recommends that the appropriate agencies of the Department of Health and Human Services (DHHS) design a model insurance-benefit package for children with asthma according to the performance measures outlined in Recommendations 1–3. This model insurance-benefit package would include a set of basic benefits for all children with asthma and certain extended benefits for children with moderate and severe persistent asthma.

Implementation Options. The National Asthma Education and Prevention Program would work with appropriate agencies in DHHS, such as the Centers for Disease Control and Prevention (CDC), the Health Care Financing Administration (HCFA), and the Health Resources and Services Administration (HRSA), to design the model asthma-benefit package. Legal experts could translate the package into contractual language. Since covered services under Medicaid are broadly defined and often subject to interpretation, it is particularly important that HCFA make explicit those model asthma benefits that are currently covered by Medicaid. State Medicaid directors could then make sure that all contracting Medicaid providers cover those services.

Funding Options. Funding for the development of asthma-specific contractual language for health care purchasers could come from a combination of public and private sources, including the CDC, HRSA, Medicaid, and health insurance associations. Asthma-related health insurance benefits would be funded through premium payments and Medicaid (see Recommendation 4). For uninsured children, these services would be funded through the public health infrastructure (see Recommendation 7).

6. Educate health care purchasers about asthma benefits

Health care purchasers can use their purchasing power to affect health care delivery patterns. They have the opportunity, through the contracting process, to change benefits or to incorporate performance measures or guarantees. The Committee recommends that, once model benefit packages for essential asthma services have been developed (see Recommendation 5), purchasers be trained in how to evaluate and procure benefit packages that encourage the provision of quality asthma care that is based on performance measures (see Recommendations 1–3).

Implementation Options. Professional and private philanthropic organizations can facilitate training of health care purchasers. The National Association of State Medicaid Directors' Maternal and Child Health Technical Advisory Group could be instrumental in educating and training state Medicaid program officers. Health-care-purchasing coalitions that have experience incorporating quality guidelines into contractual agreements could also play an important role.

Funding Options. Philanthropic organizations could fund the education process. Health insurance organizations and employers could pay for the training and technical assistance they receive, which will benefit them financially in the long run.

RECOMMENDATIONS FOR IMPROVING THE PUBLIC HEALTH INFRASTRUCTURE

7. Establish public health grants to foster* asthma-friendly *communities and home environments

The Children's Health Act of 2000 established asthma as a specific focus within the Public Health Service Act and authorized appropriation of funds to increase access to treatment and prevention in high-risk communities and to improve asthma surveillance. If adequately funded, the legislation could provide high-risk communities with resources to improve services and coordinate activities.

The Committee recommends that Congress and the Department of Health and Human Services (DHHS) work together to ensure adequate funding and implementation of the Children's Health Act, to support essential childhood asthma services (see Recommendations 1–3) to children who fall outside the health insurance system and promote *asthma-friendly* communities by addressing key environmental risk factors.

The Committee also recommends that the Secretary of DHHS consider giving states incentives to adopt policies that address environmental risk factors for asthma. For example, states could receive incentive payments if they designate smoke-free areas where housing units are close together.

Finally, the Committee recommends that Congress also supplement funds available under the Act to give states resources to use for ambulatory and school health services, with emphasis on medically underserved communities with uninsured children.

Implementation Options. Because they affect so many policy sectors, these proposed strategies for implementing the Children's Health Act of 2000 would be established in consultation with representatives from state and local housing authorities, state and local school boards, small-business regulatory agencies, patient advocacy groups, the Department of Housing and Urban Development (HUD), the Environmental Protection Agency (EPA), and DHHS.

Funding Options. Funding for *asthma-friendly* communities would come from congressional appropriations for the Children's Health Act of 2000 and from expanded Medicaid funds to provide ambulatory health care in underserved communities. Additional funds could come through appropriations for targeted programs (for example, HUD's Healthy Homes Initiative, EPA), as well as from tobacco tax revenues.

8. Promote* asthma-friendly *schools and school-based asthma programs

Asthma is the leading chronic illness–related cause of school absenteeism. Under federal law, children have legal rights to a school environment that makes an appropriate education possible.

The Committee recommends that the Department of Health and Human Services and the Department of Education, in collaboration with state and local agencies and national asthma organizations, establish performance measures for comprehensive and coordinated school health programs according to the recommendations of the National Asthma Education and Prevention Program (NAEPP).

These measures would address assessment and initial treatment of acute symptoms that occur at school, access to medications and delivery mechanisms during school hours, self-management education tailored to the school environment, links with case-management services, and evaluation of children's ability to participate in physical education, as well as support for them to do so. School nurses and personnel would be educated about performance standards of care and applicable laws. Parents of children with asthma need to know the services to which their children are entitled. School administrators and boards of education would be educated about potential liabilities for not providing school asthma services and about the revenue losses associated with asthma-related absences, and they would be given successful models for policies and practices.

Implementation Options. The Department of Health and Human Services, the Department of Education, and the NAEPP would develop the school asthma performance measures, and would coordinate activities and dissemination through the appropriate health and school national professional groups. Community-based groups would educate parents about their children's rights and school officials about legal requirements.

Funding Options. Congress could make funds available to the relevant federal departments for asthma-related school services through the Children's Health Act of 2000 or other legislation. Medicaid could cover some nurse services. Ideally, however, school-based services would be covered as a community benefit available to all children who attend school and would be financed through local or other taxes.

9. Launch a national asthma public education campaign

The Committee recommends that the Department of Health and Human Services (DHHS), in collaboration with the National Asthma Education and Prevention Program (NAEPP), national professional organizations, and state and private agencies, develop a national asthma public education campaign to increase community awareness of asthma and help children and their families recognize asthma symptoms. The Surgeon General would be the spokesperson for this campaign.

Implementation Options. The NAEPP could expand its current public education efforts and draw on media and asthma experts to design a national media campaign. These efforts could emphasize helping local community media to adapt national messages and would build on ongoing efforts by the NAEPP, the Environmental Protection Agency, the Ad Council, and others.

Funding Options. The media campaign could be partially funded by congressional appropriations to DHHS. Additional funding could come from philanthropic organizations and pharmaceutical companies. Network broadcasting companies could be asked to donate airtime.

10. Develop a national asthma surveillance system

National data about asthma are fragmented and inadequate for developing prevention, treatment, and management strategies. Therefore, the Committee recommends that the federal government spearhead creation of a national population-based asthma surveillance system to assess the magnitude and nature of the childhood asthma crisis, and that the Centers for Disease Control and Prevention (CDC) establish standards for surveillance, and fund state and local asthma surveillance units to carry out standard-driven activities, including identifying appropriate sentinel events and assessing risk factors in communities with outcomes worse than average.

Implementation Options. The CDC would take the lead in establishing standards, coordinating with other federal agencies and state health departments. For example, asthma-related data already being collected from the National Center for Health Statistics and the Health Care Financing Administration would be incorporated into the surveillance system. Health care providers and state health departments could collaborate on implementing a reporting mechanism that includes a system for appropriate medical follow-up.

Funding Options. Funding for a national asthma surveillance system would be allocated by Congress. Provisions for such funding are included in Subtitle D of the Children's Health Act of 2000. State and local communities might also provide resources, possibly assisted by matching funds from federal and state sources, respectively.

11. Develop and implement a national agenda for asthma prevention research

Although basic science research should continue at its current pace, a significant boost in funding of asthma research in humans in their natural settings is necessary to investigate and identify the possible environmental, genetic, lifestyle, and health care system factors associated with increases in asthma prevalence and morbidity.

The Committee recommends that the Department of Health and Human Services (DHHS), in collaboration with federal and state health and environmental agencies, develop and implement a national agenda for asthma prevention research, emphasizing epidemiologic, clinical, social, and behavioral sciences. Special attention would be given to reasons for disparities in asthma-related outcomes among subgroups of the population.

Implementation Options. The research agenda would be developed by DHHS, in collaboration with relevant professional and philanthropic organizations. Active and prominent interdisciplinary asthma researchers would also consult in this process.

Funding Options. The agenda would be funded through continued congressional appropriations to federal research agencies within DHHS. Specifically, additional National Institutes of Health funds would be directed to clinical, epidemiological, social, behavioral, and health services research. Additional funds could also be solicited from the pharmaceutical industry and from other private organizations.

The preceding 11 policy recommendations are mapped to the six related policy goals, funding options, and intervention sectors, in Table ES.1. A quick glance down a column reveals the comprehensiveness or specificity of a recommendation.

Taking the next step

If fully adopted, these recommendations would bring about major improvements in childhood asthma outcomes and increase the number of *asthma-friendly* communities nationwide. These policy actions can be adopted in stages and over time. The congressional attention provided by passage of the Children's Health Act of 2000 creates momentum for putting into place the kind of national childhood policy agenda described here.

The country cannot afford to wait to take action. Too many children with asthma are unnecessarily impaired. Much of the money spent on asthma is for high-cost health care services for hospitalizations and emergency visits to treat acute periods of illness. Many asthma attacks could be avoided—and much suffering prevented and many medical costs saved—if more children received good-quality, ongoing asthma care and if their communities were more *asthma-friendly*.

Table ES.1

Summary Map of Policy Recommendations

	Health Care Delivery and Financing						Public Health Infrastructure				
	Quality of Care Performance Measures			Coverage & Benefit Design			Uninsured Community and Health Services		Public Aware-ness	Surveillance and Research	
	1	2	3	4	5	6	7	8	9	10	11
Related policy goals											
Improve health care	✔	✔	✔	✔	✔	✔	✔	✔		✔	✔
Improve asthma awareness	✔	✔	✔	✔	✔	✔	✔	✔	✔	✔	✔
Ensure *asthma-friendly* schools		✔	✔		✔		✔	✔	✔		✔
Promote *asthma-safe* home environments			✔		✔		✔		✔	✔	✔
Reduce disparities	✔	✔	✔	✔	✔	✔	✔	✔	✔	✔	✔
Promote innovation	✔		✔			✔	✔	✔		✔	✔
Funding options											
Public (federal/state/local)						✔	✔			✔	✔
Both public and private	✔	✔	✔	✔	✔	✔		✔	✔		
Intervention sector(s)											
Health care system	✔	✔	✔	✔	✔	✔	✔	✔	✔	✔	✔
Education system		✔	✔				✔	✔	✔	✔	✔
Social services			✔		✔		✔	✔	✔		✔
Environmental			✔		✔		✔	✔	✔	✔	✔

NOTE:

1 = Develop and implement primary care performance measures for childhood asthma care.

2 = Teach all children with persistent asthma and their families a specific set of self-management skills.

3 = Provide case-management to high-risk children.

4 = Extend continuous health insurance coverage to all uninsured children.

5 = Develop model benefit packages for essential childhood asthma services.

6 = Educate health care purchasers about asthma benefits.

7 = Establish public health grants to foster *asthma-friendly* communities and home environments.

8 = Promote *asthma-friendly* schools and school-based asthma programs.

9 = Launch a national asthma public education campaign.

10 = Develop a national asthma surveillance system.

11 = Develop and implement a national agenda for asthma prevention research.

ACKNOWLEDGMENTS

RAND Health wishes to acknowledge the many individuals and organizations who contributed to this project.

The National Expert Committee who participated in the process provided unique insight and leadership. We would like to profusely thank each of the committee members—Noreen Clark, Nicole Lurie, Thomas Platts-Mills, Vernon Smith, and Lani Wheeler—for their expertise and enthusiasm throughout the project. We would especially like to acknowledge the essential contributions of the Co-Chairs, Steve Redd and Kevin Weiss, and the policy insight provided by Sara Rosenbaum.

We would also like to thank the 28 national organizations (listed on pages vii through x) who voluntarily reviewed the policy recommendations presented in this report. The feedback they provided to the process was indispensable.

At RAND, the authors would like to thank Marian Branch, Paul Butler, Linda Escalante, Yasmin Facey, Dennis Flieder, Shirley Hall, Carrie Imai, Christopher Kelly, Gwen Parker, Sandy Petitjean, Alaida Rodríguez, and Mary Wrazen. At the expert committee member institutions, we acknowledge the unflagging help and patience of Leslie Boss, Jo Diaz, Lenora Holland, Jay Inglis, Sylvia Koski, Tammy Rowe, Maria Sandoval, and Robin Wagner.

This project would not have been possible without the generous support of the Robert Wood Johnson Foundation. Particularly, we are deeply indebted to Seth Emont for his vision in launching this project and the Robert Wood Johnson Pediatric Asthma Initiative of which it is part. At Robert Wood Johnson, we would also like to thank Doriane Miller, Sara Thier, Paul Tarini, Liisa Rand, Sherry DeMarchi, and Phyllis Kane.

I also want to express my utmost gratitude to the RAND Health staff who contributed to this project and its completion. The skill and dedication of Will Nicholas, Sally Morton, Mary E. Vaiana, Barbara Genovese, and Carolyn Rogers were paramount. Gary Rachelefsky's expert guidance and enthusiasm were crucial throughout.

Finally, I would like to deeply thank my husband, Richard Greenberg, and Robert Brook, my mentor and Director of RAND Health, for their unwavering support of this and multiple other projects.

Marielena Lara, Principal Investigator

ABBREVIATIONS

AAAAI	American Academy of Allergy, Asthma and Immunology
AAFA	Asthma and Allergy Foundation of America
AAFP	American Academy of Family Physicians
AAHP	American Association of Health Plans
AANMA	Allergy and Asthma Network/Mothers of Asthmatics
AAP	American Academy of Pediatrics
ACAAI	American College of Allergy, Asthma, and Immunology
ACEP	American College of Emergency Physicians
AHRQ	Agency for Healthcare Research and Quality
ALA	American Lung Association
APhA	American Pharmaceutical Association
ATS	American Thoracic Society
CDC	Centers for Disease Control and Prevention
DHHS	Department of Health and Human Services
ED	Emergency Department(s)
EPA	Environmental Protection Agency

HCFA	Health Care Financing Administration
HEDIS	Health Plan Employer Data and Information Set
HHI	Healthy Homes Initiative
HIAA	Health Insurance Association of America
HRSA	Health Resources and Services Administration
HUD	Department of Housing and Urban Development
NAEPP	National Asthma Education and Prevention Program
NCHS	National Center for Health Statistics
NCQA	National Committee for Quality Assurance
NHLBI	National Heart, Lung and Blood Institute
NIAID	National Institute of Allergy and Infectious Diseases
NIEHS	National Institute of Environmental Health Sciences
NIH	National Institutes of Health
PHS	Public Health Service
SCHIP	State Children's Health Insurance Program

Chapter One

INTRODUCTION

This project was inspired by the story of one of our own patients:

Fabiola is a bright, active teenager: a good student, a cheerleader, and a member of the school choir. She is also one of an estimated 5 million American children under age 15 with asthma. Although asthma is a treatable and manageable disease, for Fabiola it was almost fatal.

Fabiola was diagnosed with asthma when she was 5. At age 10, she was referred to the county asthma clinic, where she was put on a regular program of preventive medication. Her symptoms improved dramatically for a while.

In the winter of 1997, Fabiola was hospitalized for asthma. Her working parents received a hospital bill for nearly $10,000. They did not qualify for Medicaid, and their employers did not offer insurance. They began paying the bill as best they could. However, as a result, they could no longer afford medications for Fabiola or regular checkups. Nor did they fully understand the importance of preventive care and medication. Clinic staff lost touch with Fabiola.

One night, about a year later, Fabiola stopped breathing. Fortunately, the paramedics arrived swiftly and were able to restore her breathing. She was transferred to an intensive care unit. At discharge, she was advised to return to the asthma clinic.

Back on aggressive preventive medication therapy, Fabiola's symptoms improved. Her family paid for her treatment, and clinic staff tried to get her insured. Since then, Fabiola's father has taken a new job that offers insurance coverage. Clinic staff were able to transfer Fabiola's care to an asthma specialist affiliated with her health plan. Fabiola is now nearly symptom-free and doing well at school.

Fabiola's story illustrates what can happen to children whose asthma goes unmanaged. Although Fabiola is doing well now, it took nearly 10 years after she was diagnosed to overcome the barriers and get her on track with an effective treatment regimen that her family could afford. Her experience is all too common.

To help children with asthma like Fabiola to lead productive and normal lives, the Robert Wood Johnson Foundation, in October 1999, funded RAND Health to outline future directions for childhood asthma policy in the United States. The purposes of this effort, conducted as a part of a broader Pediatric Asthma Initiative sponsored by the Foundation, were to

- Identify a range of policy actions in both the public and private sectors that could improve childhood asthma outcomes nationwide
- Select a subset of policies to create a blueprint for national policy in this area
- Outline alternatives to implement these policies that build on prior efforts.

This report summarizes our findings and recommendations. *Policy Context* provides the background for this national public health problem and a brief summary of national activities to date in this area. *Overview of Methods* describes how we engaged an interdisciplinary panel of nationally recognized leaders in childhood asthma in a structured group process to identify the 11 policy recommendations presented later in the report. *Policy Framework* outlines the comprehensive policy framework that maps the identified recommendations to one overall policy objective—to promote the development and maintenance of *asthma-friendly* communities (communities in which children are swiftly diagnosed, receive appropriate and ongoing treatment, and are not exposed to environmental factors that exacerbate their condition)—and six interrelated policy goals to meet this policy objective:

- **Improve access to and quality of asthma health care services.**
- **Improve asthma awareness among affected individuals and the general public.**
- **Ensure *asthma-friendly* schools.**
- **Promote *asthma-safe* home environments.**
- **Encourage innovation in asthma prevention and management.**
- **Reduce socioeconomic disparities in childhood asthma outcomes.**

Policy Recommendations presents the 11 policy recommendations by the following areas:

- **Improving health care delivery and financing, by**
  - — Promoting quality of care for key childhood asthma care services (Recommendations 1, 2, and 3).
  - — Expanding insurance coverage and improving benefits design (Recommendations 4 and 5).
  - — Educating health care purchasers about asthma benefits (Recommendation 6).
- **Strengthening the public health infrastructure, by**
  - — Publicly funding asthma-related services that fall outside the health insurance system (Recommendations 7 and 8).
  - — Increasing public awareness and knowledge of asthma (Recommendation 9).
  - — Improving surveillance and prevention research efforts (Recommendations 10 and 11).

Each recommendation is preceded by a brief context and justification based on available evidence and expert judgment. Each recommendation has a subsection for implementation options and funding options, outlining specific alternatives for implementing the policies. The alternatives build on prior efforts. The implementation subsection describes sectors that would be involved in implementing the recommendation (health care, education, social services, and environmental); the funding subsection discusses possible funding sources (public and/or private).

Finally, *Conclusion* summarizes the implications of the report and possible next steps in its implementation.

Chapter Two

POLICY CONTEXT

Almost everyone knows a child with asthma. Although asthma is a treatable disease, too many children with asthma suffer unnecessarily. Some even die. Yet children whose asthma is properly controlled can lead a fully active life with minimal symptoms.

Childhood asthma is a national public health problem that challenges not only the entire health system but also school systems and the many public and private organizations that track the effects of this illness, provide education and other community-based programs, and fund research into the causes of asthma. To combat this problem, improved coordination of ongoing national efforts and a significant commitment of national resources are necessary. Equally important is the commitment of individual state and local organizations and individual communities nationwide. Success will depend on the integration of local, state, and national efforts.

THE CHILDHOOD ASTHMA EPIDEMIC

The magnitude and rate of increase of asthma in this country are of epidemic proportions. The number of people in the United States with asthma has doubled in the past 15 years, to an estimated 15 million.[1] Children are the most affected: The number of asthma cases in children under age 5 years increased more than 160 percent between 1980 and 1994, and 74 percent for children ages 5 through 14 years.[2] All together, an estimated 5 million American children have this disease.[3] Although all children are affected, children who are poor, African American, or Puerto Rican suffer the most.[4-8]

THE COSTS OF ASTHMA

The costs of asthma to children with the illness, to their families, and to American society are immense. A child with uncontrolled asthma experiences symptoms that can be life-threatening and that can profoundly affect all aspects of his or her life. Children with asthma miss school frequently (an estimated 11.8 million school days per year nationwide, based on 1994 estimates).[9] These absences impede not only children's education and learning but also their parents' ability to work and support them adequately.

In 1985, asthma cost the United States an estimated $4.5 billion dollars: $2.4 billion for direct medical expenditures and $2.1 billion for indirect costs associated with school and work days lost, and premature mortality.[10] Over the ensuing decade, these costs increased to a total of $10.7 billion in 1994.[9] The Pew Environmental Health Commission predicts that total asthma annual costs could rise to $18 billion by 2020.[11] A large share of the direct costs is borne by public funds, most notably the federal, state, and local dollars that pay for Medicaid.

A significant portion of national asthma costs derives from use of high-cost health care services for *tertiary care*—hospitalizations and emergency department visits to treat acute periods of illness. Using the most recent available (1993–1995) national data, the U.S. Centers for Disease Control and Prevention (CDC) estimated that asthma accounted for 466,000 hospitalizations and 1.9 million emergency department visits per year. The corresponding figures for children under 15 years were 164,000 hospitalizations and 570,000 emergency department visits.[2]

A PUBLIC HEALTH PROBLEM WITH MULTIPLE CAUSES, REQUIRING A VARIETY OF RESPONSES

Paradoxically, the asthma epidemic coincides with significant improvements in the medical treatments available for asthma. Good primary health care delivered by a trained professional can help children with asthma lead full and active lives and prevent emergency room visits and hospitalizations.[12] Yet, in the United States today, too many children with asthma are unnecessarily impaired, and too much of what is spent on asthma is for tertiary care.

Why does this happen? The answer is complex, but there are two important reasons. First, not enough is known about what causes the disease and what factors are associated with its progression. Second, existing scientific evidence points toward multiple causes of asthma and, thus, a need for solutions that involve many different individuals and organizations. These solutions must aim not only at improving the quality of asthma care but also at modifying the physical and social environments in which children with asthma live.

Risk Factors

Research has identified several risk factors associated with the development of asthma (*incidence*) and/or its progression, persistence, and worsening (*prevalence* and *exacerbation*):

- A genetic or biologic predisposition
- Certain physical environmental exposures that may interact with a genetic predisposition[13, 14]
- Socioeconomic risk factors, including poverty and family psychosocial stressors[5, 6]
- Fragmented and inappropriate health care services.[1, 6, 7]

Socioeconomic factors are associated with heightened risk for numerous health conditions and disabilities. Despite a reduction in childhood poverty in recent years, the disparities in asthma risk have persisted. Furthermore, the proportion of children who are poor remains more than 50 percent higher than for other populations.[15]

Performance Measures for Asthma Care

Research has shown that not all asthma care is provided in accordance with national guideline recommendations.[12, 16-19] Many children with asthma and their caregivers do not use preventive medications or know how to prevent and treat asthma attacks.[20-26] Barriers to effective management of asthma include the following:

- The complexity of treating the disease (multiple medications and a variety of equipment needs)

- The costs of care stemming from lack of health insurance or gaps in coverage
- The lack of comprehensive performance measures and broad implementation strategies to improve and strengthen the quality of provider performance.

Randomized control trials of case-management services and other quality improvement strategies[27-29] indicate that improved access to quality care for asthma can reduce childhood asthma morbidity and reduce associated tertiary health care utilization.

Environmental Factors

Growing evidence suggests that if the long-term goal is to reduce asthma severity, improving the accessibility and quality of health care delivery may not be sufficient. Certain indoor environmental exposures, including tobacco smoke, cat hair, dust mites, and cockroaches, have been shown to make asthma worse. Thus, environmental control is indispensable for sensitive individuals.[1, 14] But the authority to identify and intervene to control physical environmental exposures does not fall within the traditional jurisdiction of the health care system. Instead, that authority belongs to government housing and environmental agencies, whose sources of funding and legal powers are separate from those of the health care system.

Effects on Schools

Childhood asthma has a significant impact on school systems. Life-threatening acute asthma symptoms can occur at school. Children with asthma often miss school and require remedial coursework, thereby further taxing schools already limited in resources. As with environmental matters, schools' legal authorities and sources of funding are separate from those in the health care system.

A Complex Problem

What we know about childhood asthma points toward a multi-dimensional policy solution that involves restructuring and coordinating efforts in many sectors of our society. The need for a multisector approach is not unique to asthma, but the financial and human consequences of not taking such an approach to asthma are particularly great. Appropriate management of asthma in children would not only reduce the symptom burden and improve the quality of life for children and their families, but would also produce significant cost savings among patients with severe disease.[30]

CURRENT ASTHMA EFFORTS NEED INCREASED COORDINATION AND FUNDING

Public-Sector Efforts

National Heart, Lung, and Blood Institute (NHLBI) and the National Asthma Education and Prevention Program (NAEPP). In 1989, NHLBI created the NAEPP, guided by a coordinating committee made up of representatives from 37 government agencies, professional organizations, and lay organizations with expertise in and commitment to improving asthma outcomes—thus, important participants in defining and solving the childhood asthma problem. The NAEPP's broad agenda to date has included activities in clinical management guidelines, clinician education, family and patient education, public education, school-based education, community-based partnership and outreach, and quality of delivery systems.[1, 12] In 1991, the NAEPP developed the *Guidelines for the Diagnosis and Management of Asthma,* which were revised in 1997[12] and widely disseminated. More recently, the NAEPP has focused on developing and sustaining asthma coalitions in high-risk communities to promote adoption of guidelines and creation of *asthma-friendly* communities at the local level.

The U.S. Department of Health and Human Service's (DHHS) *Action Against Asthma* and Other Federal Efforts. Multiple federal agencies (NHLBI, National Institute of Allergy and Infectious Diseases [NIAID], National Institute of Environmental Health Sciences [NIEHS], Agency for Healthcare Research and Quality [AHRQ], Centers for Disease Control and Prevention [CDC], Environmental Protection Agency [EPA]) are conducting or providing support for research, tracking the impact of the disease and its possible risk factors (CDC, EPA), and providing or paying for health care and social services in poor and otherwise underserved asthma populations

(Medicaid/Health Care Financing Administration, Health Resources and Services Administration, Head Start, Department of Housing and Urban Development). For example, NIAID and NIEHS support several asthma research programs, including the Inner-City Asthma Study and the Home Endotoxin and Childhood Asthma Program. The Agency for Healthcare Research and Quality and the Blue Cross/Blue Shield Evidence-based Practice Center are conducting a systematic review of asthma evidence. The EPA has a multi-component educational program emphasizing recognition and control of asthma environmental triggers, including incorporation of environmental controls in standards for clinical practice; school-based, daycare-based, and in-home education; smoking-cessation programs; development and implementation of the *Indoor Air Quality Tools for Schools*[31]; and an asthma media campaign in collaboration with the Ad Council.

Prior and ongoing federal efforts, including the asthma workgroup of the President's Taskforce on Environmental Risks and Safety for Children and the *Healthy People 2010* objectives for asthma,[32] have also provided leadership and vision in this area. In May 2000, the Department of Health and Human Services released *Action Against Asthma*, a catalogue of asthma-related federal efforts to date and a strategic plan for future federal efforts in this area.[1] *Action Against Asthma* outlines 22 priority strategies in four general areas for DHHS investment over the next five years; each strategy is described in terms of two to four specific activities or actions to be carried out by DHHS agencies.

Federal Spending in Asthma. During fiscal year 1999, DHHS spent $145 million in asthma research and less than $10 million on the public health practice of asthma. The federal government also spent an estimated $1 billion in asthma-related treatment costs.[1]

The Department of Health and Human Service's funding for asthma in fiscal year 2000 was increased to $183 million. Yet this total appears to be extremely limited in view of both the five-year agenda proposed in *Action Against Asthma* and the country's estimated total annual $11 billion in costs for asthma.[1, 10] In addition, most asthma discretionary spending has been earmarked for research rather than for improving the public health practice of asthma. Although epidemiological, behavioral, health services, and other prevention research is currently being funded, most research dollars are currently spent in basic science research.[1]

This research has led to improved understanding of the pathophysiology of the disease and to remarkable improvements in asthma care. However, implementation of these improvements is highly variable, and selected geographic areas and subpopulations carry a disproportionate burden of disease. It is time now to increase funding for translational research that includes these high-risk populations, and to invest in an improved public health infrastructure to ensure widespread availability of quality asthma care.

Private-Sector Efforts

Many asthma-related activities occur under the auspices of private-sector organizations, such as professional societies, private insurance and managed care companies, private school systems, the pharmaceutical industry, lay voluntary organizations, and private philanthropy.

For example, lay organizations play an important role in education and advocacy. The American Lung Association developed *Action on Asthma*,[33] an advocacy manual for the development and implementation of state and local policies related to asthma. The Asthma and Allergy Foundation of America supported and disseminated a study on the increasing costs of asthma in America and in specific states[34] and provides training and coordination of patient support groups around the country. The Allergy and Asthma Network/Mothers of Asthmatics has numerous publications and newsletters educating families about asthma and has developed the *2000 Report Card on Asthma*, which grades the nation's progress according to several important indicators.[35]

Professional societies have played key roles in translating and disseminating national asthma guidelines to their constituents. For example, the American Academy of Allergy, Asthma and Immunology (AAAAI) has supported the development of the user-friendly pediatric asthma guide based on the 1997 NHLBI guidelines,[36] continuing medical education (CME) courses for primary care professionals, patient education courses and materials, and websites for professionals, patients, and the public. In July 1999, the AAAAI, in conjunction with the American Association of Health Plans, also created "Taking on Asthma"—a national program to bring health plans and health professionals together. The American Association of Family Physicians also has sponsored CME courses and has selected asthma as its clinical focus in 2000–2001. The American College of Chest Physicians developed asthma pocket cards for professionals according to the 1997 guidelines. The American College of Emergency Physicians and the Society for Academic Emergency Medicine are involved in important activities, including efforts to eliminate barriers to insurance coverage for all children and interventions involving the emergency department setting. The American Pharmaceutical Association and its Foundation have supported demonstration projects to improve asthma care, capitalizing on the key role of the community pharmacist in working directly with patients with asthma.

The Robert Wood Johnson Foundation, in addition to being an active participant in some of these private efforts, launched its own Pediatric Asthma Initiative in 1999. The purpose of this initiative is to address current gaps in national childhood asthma care through clinical and nonclinical approaches to improving the management of childhood asthma. The ultimate goal of the initiative is to reduce emergency department visits, hospital admissions, and costs caused by poorly managed asthma. To achieve these goals, six separate but related programs have been supported: (1) demonstration programs utilizing evidence-based clinical care models for Medicaid managed care populations; (2) demonstration programs for childhood asthma management in emergency departments; (3) development of a brief intervention for providers; (4) exploration of barriers to financing and treatment; (5) community-based efforts to improve access to and quality of medical services; and (6) identification of policies that could improve childhood asthma outcomes (summarized in this report).

Other independent, nonprofit organizations provide important information to consumers and health care providers and purchasers. For example, the National Committee for Quality Assurance is an independent, nonprofit organization whose mission is to evaluate and report on the quality of the nation's managed care organizations. Its Asthma Measurement Advisory Panel has been developing measures for the performance of health care organizations on several aspects of asthma care.[37] However, these measures emphasize short-term outcomes and are not easily translated to non–managed care populations. Furthermore, lack of financial support for performance measure development has hindered progress.

Although these and other private efforts are very valuable, they are not yet integrated comprehensive public policies. Private organizations on the NAEPP Coordinating Committee have succeeded in creating partnerships among public- and private-sector activities; yet, even more collaboration will be necessary for developing and implementing the concerted and comprehensive childhood asthma policy agenda required to accomplish the objective of *asthma-friendly* communities nationwide.

Chapter Three

OVERVIEW OF METHODS

Because many factors affect asthma and its management, a multi-strategy policy approach is needed to improve childhood asthma outcomes. To develop specific recommendations, we used both a structured panel meeting and policy formulation methods. The paucity of evidence on the potential impact of policies in key areas meant that interdisciplinary expert judgment had to be substituted in some instances.

We used a nominal group method to structure the expert judgment process. This method is described in detail elsewhere[38] and has been used previously in policy exercises.[39] In general, this method entailed

- Selecting and convening an interdisciplinary group of asthma and policy experts
- Identifying policy actions that would lead to improvement of national childhood asthma outcomes
- Soliciting ratings, via mail, of the policy actions we identified, prior to the expert panel meeting
- Analyzing the ratings
- Using the analysis to guide discussion at a face-to-face meeting of the panel
- Selecting the final policy recommendations by anonymous voting during the panel meeting

- Having the expert panel and a broad set of external organizations extensively review the final report.

The panel of experts was led by two chairs of national prominence who have first-hand experience with the economic and policy issues of asthma, and current or prior clinical experience. We completed the panel by selecting an interdisciplinary group of six additional individuals with expertise in asthma education and community outreach, delivery of asthma health care services in different settings, environmental assessment and control, epidemiology and surveillance, health care financing, and government programs and policy.

From a review of publications familiar to the RAND staff and expert panel and discussion among the RAND project team, we identified a preliminary list of policy actions. We revised this list on the basis of comments and suggestions from the panel, and circulated it via mail to the panel.

As part of the pre-meeting voting exercise, panelists were asked to rate the priority of possible policy recommendations according to predetermined criteria:

- Feasibility of implementation
- Whether supported by research or historical evidence
- Reduction of inequalities in asthma outcomes among underserved children
- Reduction of net societal costs for asthma, including the costs for implementation
- Improvement of global pediatric health-related outcomes, including improved child and family quality-of-life and reduced symptom burden and preventable hospitalizations and deaths.

Panelists were asked to rate each policy action on a four-point scale for each criterion, as well as to provide an overall grade. We analyzed the data and used an algorithm determined *a priori* to determine the top set of candidate recommendations (those that were in the top 20 in overall grade, and that scored in the top two-thirds on all five criteria).

The face-to-face panel meeting followed a predetermined agenda and repeated voting exercises. The meeting began with a debate on the candidate recommendations that met the algorithm criteria, as well as those that did not. Based on candidate recommendations in this first round of discussion, 21 policy recommendations, consisting of some rewordings of the original policy actions as well as some collapsing of policy actions into a single recommendation, were subjected to a vote. This vote, along with some additional discussion, resulted in the final set of 11 policy recommendations to be included in the policy blueprint. The final set of policy recommendations was drafted by RAND staff, reviewed and approved by members of the committee of experts, and sent for comment to the 28 organizations that are listed as external reviewers of this report. Based on the feedback, suggested modifications of the policy recommendations were reviewed by committee members through a repeat voting process.

(For more details on how the national expert committee was chosen and how a set of candidate policy options was generated, reviewed, and selected, please refer to the accompanying methods report, RAND MR-1330/1-RWJ. That report also discusses in more detail the pre-meeting and in-meeting voting exercises and post-meeting review activities.[38])

During the period in which the Committee carried out its deliberations and policy development activities, March–September 2000, Congress considered and enacted legislation pertinent to childhood asthma. To ensure that the Committee's recommendations appropriately accounted for this new spending authority, we analyzed all asthma-related legislation—a total of 32 separate pieces—using standard legislative research techniques. The Children's Health Act of 2000 was analyzed in greater depth. (For more details about the methodology and a fuller analysis of the Act, see the Appendix.)

Chapter Four

POLICY FRAMEWORK

The expert process described above led to the conclusion that a successful national childhood asthma policy agenda should have national, state, and community components and be comprehensive.

PROMOTION OF *ASTHMA-FRIENDLY* COMMUNITIES NATIONWIDE

Communities are the ultimate focus for asthma-related policy efforts, because it is at the community level that children with asthma and their caregivers interact with and obtain services from the health care system, schools, and other important social institutions. Community-based and community-centered efforts thus are the essential cornerstone of a public health approach to the problem. Consequently, all national policies (both public and private) should be considered with an eye toward the promotion of *asthma-friendly* communities nationwide.

An *asthma-friendly community* is one in which children with asthma are swiftly diagnosed, receive appropriate and ongoing treatment, and are not exposed to environmental factors that exacerbate their condition. *Asthma-friendly communities* have health care, school, and social agencies that are *prepared* and *able to respond to* the interdisciplinary needs of children with asthma and their families. *Asthma-friendly communities* ensure *safe* and *protected* surroundings (including their homes) that minimize children's exposures to physical and social environmental risks that worsen their disease. In *asthma-friendly communities*, public awareness messages demonstrate an understanding of children with asthma and their families.

COMPREHENSIVE POLICY GOALS AND APPROACHES

Because many factors affect asthma treatment and shape approaches to management, a national childhood asthma policy agenda needs to be comprehensive. Comprehensive refers, first, to the interdisciplinary nature and wide range of policy goals and tools that are necessary to meet the overall policy objective of *asthma-friendly* communities. Comprehensive also means collaboration among the health care, education, environmental, and other social sectors of our society traditionally supported by different funding. Finally, comprehensive implies participation of both the public and private sectors and integration of public health activities across local, state, and federal levels. Without enactment and coordination of policies across all sectors, successful childhood asthma control and management will not be possible.

POLICY GOALS EMERGING FROM THE EXPERT PANEL PROCESS

Policy Goal No. 1: Improve Access to and Quality of Asthma Health Care Services

Because appropriate medical care can control asthma symptoms,[1, 12, 36] a child's capacity to lead a normal life is highly related to the accessibility of high-quality health services. Indicators of access to care include the absence of barriers to care, such as lack of health insurance coverage, and the availability and use of asthma services and medications when the child needs them.[25, 40]

Quality of care refers to what actually happens when the child and family interact with the health care system (process of care), the health care system's structural capacity to provide optimal care, and the effect that health care services have on patient health and quality-of-life outcomes.[25] For example, *good quality* means receiving care from a provider who is accessible in accordance with need and residence, is able to communicate effectively with the patient and family, and practices according to the latest evidence-based guidelines for effective medical management and patient education. Having access to health services does not necessarily ensure that care is of optimal quality. Thus, improving *both* access and quality of services should be the goal of a comprehensive effort; possible differences in how proposed approaches may affect access and quality of services should be part of assessing those approaches.

Policy Goal No. 2: Improve Asthma Awareness Among Affected Individuals and the General Public

Scientific evidence and clinical experience document both the effectiveness and the necessity of patient self-management strategies to control asthma.[12, 36, 41] The effectiveness of patient self-management depends on the child's and family's familiarity with asthma symptoms and their capacity, knowledge, and motivation to adopt effective prevention and management strategies.

Improving the general public's awareness about asthma is also important. Public understanding can promote the capacity of lay people who interact with children to recognize asthma, thereby increasing chances of early referral and minimizing the risks posed by potentially life-threatening situations when they occur. Drawing attention to asthma and its consequences also can promote collaboration among the health care, environmental, education, and social service sectors, advocacy efforts, and policymakers. Other countries, such as Australia, have experience in controlling childhood asthma through strategies that improve general public awareness of the condition.[42]

Policy Goal No. 3: Ensure *Asthma-Friendly* Schools

A school's *asthma-friendliness* refers to its capacity to promote quality-of-life for children with asthma, through policies and facilities that support and encourage adequate knowledge, time, and commitment of school staff to meet the needs of children with asthma during school hours and in after-school facilities.[43] Schools are a natural community hub for children and families, and thus a good base for asthma education and referral to health care and social services.

Furthermore, ensuring school *asthma-friendliness* would likely benefit all children attending school. The additional time and resources devoted to this end would likely promote the school's focus on the health and well-being of all school children. For example, additional emphasis on the participation of children with asthma in sports and exercise could lead to increased physical activity for all children during school hours.

Nevertheless, the time and resources spent in asthma-specific programs need to be carefully balanced against potential costs. These costs include the possible decreased attention by school nurses and other personnel to children without asthma and the possible loss of valuable student class time (in the case of asthma programs incorporated into the general curriculum). Thus, the cost-effectiveness of alternative school models needs to be evaluated.

Policy Goal No. 4: Promote *Asthma-Safe* Home Environments

Both scientific evidence and expert consensus suggest that exposure to indoor allergens and irritants can exacerbate asthma symptoms among sensitive individuals, and may play a role in the development of asthma.[14, 44] Because many parents fear for their children's safety, children may be spending increasing amounts of time inside their homes. Policies that promote *asthma-safe* home environments would involve eliminating or controlling asthma-provoking allergens and irritants through collaboration among families, housing authorities, and payers.

Policy Goal No. 5: Encourage Innovation in Asthma Prevention and Management

Although asthma's causes are still not fully understood, great strides in treatment and management strategies allow people with asthma to lead normal and productive lives. But the capacity to improve the treatment, management, and control of asthma will also require advancing medical knowledge about asthma treatment and evaluating new strategies—such as environmental modification, immunological intervention, and lifestyle changes—for preventing and managing symptoms. More research on quality improvement and other strategies to improve health care delivery systems is also necessary.

Policy Goal No. 6: Reduce Socioeconomic Disparities in Childhood Asthma Outcomes

The greater burden of the asthma epidemic among low-income, minority, and other underserved populations is extensively documented and is a widely recognized national public health problem.[1] Low-income children are more likely to suffer the burden of disease[45] and less likely to have the resources to adequately address the impact of illness. Despite improvements in insurance coverage in recent years,[46] some 10 million children remain uninsured and may not receive needed health care services. Low-income children are significantly more likely to dwell in substandard housing and are much more likely to reside in communities with environmental risk factors that exacerbate asthma. Among all low-income children, minority children may be the most likely to be at risk, because they are disproportionately likely to live in high-poverty central-city communities with high levels of pollutants and poor housing stock. Reducing these disparities will require efforts that promote all of the policy goals outlined above while simultaneously paying special attention to these populations. Without this focused attention, the special needs of these populations may not be met, and the gap in asthma care outcomes associated with socioeconomic disparities may widen.

Chapter Five

POLICY RECOMMENDATIONS

The 11 policy recommendations fall into two major categories—"Improving Health Care Delivery and Financing" and "Strengthening the Public Health Infrastructure." Each category and its related subcategories are described before the corresponding policy recommendations are presented.

IMPROVING HEALTH CARE DELIVERY AND FINANCING

The six recommendations in this category are designed to improve the quality of asthma-related health care services and to increase access to these services through expansions in insurance coverage and improvements in the benefit structures of public and private insurance. Directed at health care providers, purchasers, and regulators, the recommendations fall into two subcategories: "Promoting Quality of Care for Key Childhood Asthma Care Services" and "Expanding Coverage and Improving Benefits Design."

Promoting Quality of Care for Key Childhood Asthma Care Services

In light of the highly decentralized nature of the American health care system and the challenges thus inherent in any effort to improve the quality of health care, the three recommendations in this subcategory focus on the promotion of quality of care in three key areas of asthma care: primary care, self-management education, and targeted case-management. Promoting quality of care includes development, dissemination, and regular updating of evidence-based standards; and implementation and maintenance of these standards through quality improvement strategies by health care regulators, purchasers, and delivery organizations.

Recommendation 1. Develop and implement primary care performance measures for childhood asthma care

Context. Delivering the highest-quality primary care available to children with asthma is a complex and resource-intensive undertaking. National policies in this area are necessary to prevent, to the extent possible, urgent treatment of uncontrolled cases in hospitals and emergency departments. However, until universal access to appropriate primary care services is improved, efforts to integrate emergency-care physicians in primary asthma management and to facilitate communication and linkages between emergency care and primary care are essential.

Evidence-based practice guidelines are available for childhood asthma care in the ambulatory setting.[12] Nonetheless, there is a substantial gap between what is accepted as best practice and what is actually implemented in the clinical setting.[16-19] This gap can be attributed to, among other factors, provider resistance to the use of guidelines, provider disagreement or lack of familiarity with guidelines, and lack of organizational support and financial incentives for guideline implementation.

Despite these barriers, there is evidence that childhood asthma guidelines are more likely to be followed than are guidelines for other conditions.[47] This willingness on the part of providers underscores the importance of efforts to continually update and disseminate clinical guidelines for primary care management of asthma. In addition, health care delivery organizations will need to create supportive organizational environments for effective guideline implementation strategies.[48-50]

1.0 The Committee recommends that:

Health care regulators, insurers, and delivery organizations use effective strategies to implement the evidence-based clinical guidelines for primary care management of childhood asthma, regularly updated and disseminated by the National Asthma Education and Prevention Program (NAEPP), to health care providers and professional organizations. Specifically, the Committee recommends that:

1.1 Evidence-based performance measures for childhood asthma primary care cover initial diagnosis and evaluation, prescription of medications and medical devices, effective patient-doctor communication, and ongoing treatment and management.

1.2 National health care quality organizations incorporate selected evidence-based performance measures into their quality monitoring systems, to promote adherence to asthma primary care guidelines.

1.3 Health care purchasers encourage adherence to asthma primary care guidelines among contracting health plans, through incentives tied to specific asthma-related performance measures.

1.4 Health care delivery organizations use guideline-implementation and provider-education strategies of proven effectiveness to support providers in their efforts to optimize performance according to specific asthma primary care measures.

1.5 Interventions designed to improve communication and coordination between emergency care and primary care management of childhood asthma be developed and evaluated.

Implementation Options. The NAEPP, in collaboration with the National Committee for Quality Assurance (NCQA), would continue to coordinate the update, review, and dissemination of childhood asthma primary care guidelines. The review of evidence would follow the Agency for Healthcare Research and Quality's evidence-based practice model and be conducted in collaboration with the appropriate professional organizations. The NAEPP guidelines would be updated, as appropriate, according to the latest report of the Blue Cross/Blue Shield Evidence-based Practice Center on the management of chronic asthma.

Guidelines would be disseminated to insurers, managed care organizations, state Medicaid and State Children's Health Insurance Program agencies, and employers and purchasers, as well as to health care providers and professional organizations. "Taking on Asthma," the program created by the American Association of Health Plans, in conjunction with the American Academy of Allergy, Asthma and Immunology (AAAAI), offers a mechanism for this dissemination. Designed specifically to develop and disseminate standardized asthma guidelines across all health plans in a given community, this program is currently in its pilot phase and may provide a coordinated dissemination model to be emulated in communities across the country. In addition, the National Association of State Medicaid Directors' Maternal and Child Health Technical Advisory Group could be instrumental in the implementation of childhood asthma guidelines and performance measures among Medicaid providers.

The NCQA and other quality monitoring organizations would work with the NAEPP and professional organizations (AAAAI, American Pharmaceutical Association [APhA], American Academy of Pediatrics [AAP], American Academy of Family Physicians [AAFP], American College of Allergy, Asthma, and Immunology [ACAAI], American College of Emergency Physicians [ACEP], and American Thoracic Society [ATS]) and other patient and voluntary organizations (the Allergy and Asthma Network/Mothers of Asthmatics, Asthma and Allergy Foundation [AAFA], and American Lung Association) to incorporate asthma-care performance measures into the Health Plan Employer Data and Information Set system or into alternative quality measurement systems in different patient settings. The work of the Health Care Financing Administration, NCQA, and the American Diabetes Association to develop a comprehensive set of diabetes performance measures could be used as a model for developing a similar set of asthma measures. These performance measures could be incorporated into contracts between health care purchasers and plans, much as are specific covered benefits (see Recommendation 6). Given the frequent lack of good clinical and administrative data to capture performance measures, special attention should be given to evaluating and refining existing data sources and developing new data sources (see Recommendation 11).

The recent work of the National Cancer Institute (reported in a personal communication with NCQA) in establishing a program supporting the dissemination of cancer guidelines could also serve as a model. The NAEPP would also continue to compile and disseminate evidence on effective guideline implementation strategies to be used by health care delivery and professional organizations. The APhA, AAAAI, AAP, AAFP, ACAAI, ACEP, and ATS would provide effective provider education programs for guideline-based asthma management. Health care purchasers and delivery organizations that have successfully implemented asthma guidelines would be asked to share their experience and expertise.

Until all children have access to appropriate primary care services for asthma, efforts could be made to educate emergency physicians, hospitalists, and other acute care practitioners in recognizing asthma (initial diagnosis) and prescribing preventive medications and medical devices. Initiatives that explore better communication between acute care practitioners and primary care providers and link acute care to primary care could be developed and tested.

Funding Options. Federal funding would support the ongoing and enlarged role of the NAEPP in maintaining up-to-date guidelines. The NAEPP could also solicit funding from private sources to supplement these activities, using an "equal-contributions-from-all" model. The NAEPP raised equal funds from a collaborative of 16 pharmaceutical firms to support the publication of its initial guidelines. Funding for performance measures could be sought from the pharmaceutical industry, HCFA, and NCQA. Funding for childhood asthma primary care services could be requested by state agencies and advocates from federal and state public and private health insurers, as described in Recommendations 4–6. Other funding for updating, reviewing, and disseminating clinical guidelines for the primary care management of childhood asthma would continue to come from the health care and health insuring organizations that currently perform these tasks.

Recommendation 2. Teach all children with persistent asthma and their families a specific set of self-management skills

Context. Since much of the daily management of asthma requires specific knowledge, problem-solving skills, and behavior change on the part of patients and their families, it is important to educate patients and their families about asthma symptoms and treatments and to train them in asthma self-management. This education and training, including follow-up, is one of the most important aspects of medical care for patients with asthma.[51, 52]

Evidence suggests that educational interventions increase patients' knowledge about asthma and improve their self-management skills.[41, 53] There is also evidence that asthma education can reduce hospitalizations and emergency department (ED) visits.[54, 55] Several studies have shown that pharmacists can be particularly effective in improving asthma-related outcomes through patient education interventions.[56-58] Since the content of education programs has tended to vary, it will be important to identify the key elements of effective programs, which can then be broadly disseminated. Furthermore, the challenges of applying the results of research to daily practice settings may be particularly great for economically disadvantaged populations.[20-29]

Ideally, all children with asthma should receive self-management education. Given limited health care resources, priority should be given to children with persistent asthma. However, all children, regardless of their clinical classification, should receive asthma self-management education upon discharge from hospitalizations and ED visits.

2.0 The Committee recommends that:

The National Asthma Education and Prevention Program (NAEPP) use its current recommendations for asthma self-management education to develop and disseminate a specific set of performance measures to be used for quality monitoring, and that health care purchasers and providers use these performance measures to encourage self-management education among all children with *persistent asthma* (defined as reported asthma symptoms more than twice a week in the absence of preventive medication[12, 36]) and their families. Specifically, the Committee recommends that:

2.1 Asthma self-management education and related written materials be evidence-based; be adapted for different patient groups to be culturally and language appropriate; meet varied literacy levels; focus on developing self-management skills and modifying behavior; and be specifically designed for patients in partnership with their families and other caretakers.

2.2 Asthma self-management education modules be developed for both the primary care setting and for targeted interventions aimed at children with both acute and persistent asthma before they are discharged for an asthma-related emergency department visit and/or hospitalization.

2.3 Health care purchasers make patient self-management education a covered and reimbursable service, when provided by a physician, pharmacist, certified health educator, or other health professional (see Recommendation 5).

2.4 Health care purchasers and delivery organizations provide incentives to health plans, providers, and patients to encourage the completion and mastery of self-management education among all children with persistent asthma and their families.

Implementation Options. The Patient and Public Education Subcommittee of the NAEPP, in collaboration with appropriate professional organizations, including the National Asthma Educator Certification Board, American Pharmaceutical Association (APhA), American Thoracic Society (ATS), and American Lung Association, would take the lead in establishing performance measures for the content of asthma education and self-management programs and in disseminating these measures. The National Committee for Quality Assurance (NCQA) and other quality monitoring organizations could work with the NAEPP to incorporate these measures into NCQA's HEDIS performance measurement system or into alternative quality monitoring systems. The APhA, ATS, American Academy of Allergy, Asthma and Immunology, American Academy of Pediatrics, American Academy of Family Physicians, American College of Allergy, Asthma and Immunology, American College of Emergency Physicians, and American Association of Health Plans would be involved in developing educational materials for patients and their families, and would work closely with their local affiliates to implement asthma patient education at the local facility level. Although children and families may be receptive to educational interventions when they are receiving acute treatment in the hospital or emergency department, these environments may have limited time and resources. These limitations should be taken into account when developing educational modules for these settings.

Funding Options. Funding for the development of performance measures would come from private philanthropic organizations, the National Heart, Lung and Blood Institute, National Institute of Allergy and Infectious Diseases, National Institute of Environmental Health Sciences, and Agency for Healthcare Research and Quality. Collaborative funding ("equal-contributions-from-all") from the pharmaceutical industry could also be sought. National efforts to disseminate educational programs could be supported by federal funds. Funding for providing asthma self-management education to patients would be covered by public and private insurers, as allowed by federal and state laws (see Recommendations 5–6). For children without health insurance, these services would be covered through the public health infrastructure (see Recommendation 7).

Recommendation 3. Provide case-management to high-risk children

Context. Children at highest risk for poor asthma outcomes can benefit from asthma case-management interventions. Broadly defined, *asthma case-management* consists of a comprehensive set of services, including intensive tracking, coordination of care, and follow-up, using available patient-tracking tools and teams of pharmacy, medical, nursing, social work, and case-management staff.[59, 60] For example, several studies have suggested that pharmacists may prove to be central members of the case-management team, given their frequent contact with patients and the centrality of proper drug dosage and administration to effective asthma management.[57, 61, 62] However, the components of case-management vary and not all interventions have been evaluated to demonstrate their relative effectiveness.

Case-management can supplement the effect of patient education (see Recommendation 2) by providing additional patient support mechanisms, particularly to high-risk children. One recent clinical trial showed that asthma education with case-management led to greater reductions in emergency department and hospital use among children with asthma than did education alone.[28] Other evidence suggests that case-management is effective in reducing morbidity and service utilization among low-income children with moderate to severe asthma.[29, 63] However, the impact of case-management alone, without education, has yet to be fully evaluated.

Given the high cost of providing case-management services, these services would be most cost-effective if focused on children of low socioeconomic status, for whom the probability of poor asthma management is higher.[20, 21, 23, 25-27, 64] High-risk children in need of case-management services can also be identified as those experiencing multiple asthma-related hospitalizations or emergency department visits, or experiencing a life-threatening event, regardless of where they live or their socioeconomic status.

3.0 The Committee recommends that:

The National Asthma Education and Prevention Program (NAEPP) develop, disseminate, and regularly update evidence-based performance measures for childhood asthma case-management, and that health care purchasers and providers promote their use among all high-risk children with asthma. Specifically, the Committee recommends that:

3.1 Asthma case-management be provided by multidisciplinary teams (pharmacists, physicians, nurses, social workers, health educators, etc.) and include asthma education (see Recommendation 2), follow-up home visits by nurses, coordination with school-based health services, home environmental assessment and control, and patient tracking through administrative and/or pharmacy data systems.

3.2 For children with multiple asthma-related hospital or emergency department visits, case-management protocols be initiated as part of the discharge process.

3.3 Health care organizations target asthma case-management services in their quality improvement efforts, and health care purchasers adequately reimburse case-management services (see Recommendation 5).

Implementation Options. To establish guidelines for effective case-management activities, the National Asthma Education and Prevention Program and the Association for Healthcare Research and Quality Asthma Evidence-based Practice Center would take the lead in synthesizing existing research on asthma case-management among children at risk for acute asthma attacks that result in high-cost care. Appropriate professional organizations (American Pharmaceutical Association, American Academy of Allergy, Asthma and Immunology, American Academy of Pediatrics, American Academy of Family Physicians, American College of Allergy, Asthma, and Immunology, American College of Emergency Physicians, and American Thoracic Society) would disseminate these guidelines to primary care providers, targeting those in high-risk areas. The American Association of Health Plans could build on current efforts in this area by determining the proportion of health plans that currently cover asthma case-management services and educating those that do not about the cost-effectiveness of providing NAEPP-recommended case-management services to high-risk patients. State Medicaid and State Children's Health Insurance Program (SCHIP) programs could ensure that all contracting health plans have the capacity to provide case-management services to their high-risk asthma patients and to furnish care in accordance with established guidelines and standards. The Health Resources and Services Administration could ensure that federally funded community health centers have the capacity to provide case-management services to their high-risk asthma patients.

Funding Options. Funding for updating, reviewing, and disseminating performance measures for childhood asthma case-management interventions would continue to come from the organizations that currently perform these tasks. Additionally, the pharmaceutical industry could provide collaborative funds following the "equal-contributions-from-all" model used by the NAEPP to fund its initial asthma guidelines. Funding for the provision of asthma case-management services would come from public and private health insurers, including Medicaid, which covers case-management services for children (see Recommendations 5–6). Certain extended services (durable medical equipment, specialty care, home health care) that are deemed uninsurable would be covered through the public health infrastructure (for example, Title V, The Public Health Service Act) (see Recommendation 7).

Expanding Coverage and Improving Benefits Design

Many studies have documented a strong link between health care insurance and children's access to primary and preventive health care.[65] But having insurance is not, by itself, sufficient. Coverage should be for the range of services included in accepted quality guidelines for asthma care, and cost-sharing through premiums, deductibles, and coinsurance must be modest enough to avoid deterring access to care.[66] The three recommendations in this subcategory address the expansion of health insurance coverage, the development of "evidence-based" benefits packages, and the education of health care purchasers and delivery organizations on how to promote evidence-based asthma care.

Recommendation 4. Extend continuous health insurance coverage to all uninsured children

Context. All children need health insurance. Access to health insurance is associated with increased use of appropriate health care services and with better health outcomes for a range of conditions, including asthma.[67, 68] Continuous insurance coverage is critical for improving the health of children with asthma.

Existing insurance mechanisms can go a long way toward achieving the goal of insuring all children. In concert, the current Medicaid and State Children's Health Insurance Program (SCHIP) have the potential to ensure that virtually all children have access to health insurance coverage, regardless of family income. Under these programs, states already have the option to cover all otherwise uninsured children whose families require subsidized public insurance for their children. Some states have chosen to cover children in families with incomes at 200 percent, 300 percent, or even 400 percent of the federal poverty level.[69] State Medicaid and SCHIP programs also have the option of providing 12 months of continuous coverage, regardless of changes in eligibility status, as well as immediate enrollment of applicants through the use of presumptive eligibility.

But even if states were to aggressively pursue coverage for lower-income children, two groups of children would still be at risk for being uninsured: (1) children in moderate-income working families who earn too much to qualify for Medicaid or SCHIP but whose employers do not offer them affordable health insurance, and (2) children who are not citizens and who, if recent arrivals, would qualify for Medicaid emergency coverage only. The 1996 Personal Responsibility and Work Opportunity Reconciliation Act, which reformed national welfare, bars SCHIP coverage for recently arrived noncitizen children who are legal residents, even for emergency care. Studies suggest that noncitizen children are the least likely of all children to have access to health insurance.[70] This coverage gap may continue to widen.[71]

4.0 The Committee recommends that:

To eliminate barriers to full coverage of all children, Congress extend continuous health insurance coverage to all children through further expansion of Medicaid and SCHIP, as well as through complementary laws creating subsidies for employer-based insurance. Specifically, the Committee recommends that:

4.1 Governors and state legislatures make maximum use of existing state Medicaid and SCHIP program options—including expanded coverage, continuous coverage, and presumptive eligibility—to extend coverage to uninsured and underinsured children.

4.2 Federal and state policies create financial incentives and subsidy arrangements that are generous enough to encourage large and small employers to offer affordable coverage to their workers with children.

4.3 Federal and state policies extend health insurance coverage to all children residing in the United States, regardless of legal status or duration of legal residency.

Implementation Options. Asthma-related professional and lay organizations would develop collaborations to educate state governments about the importance of improving Medicaid and SCHIP coverage, as well as the importance of new laws that encourage employers to furnish affordable coverage. Health insurance organizations, such as the Health Insurance Association of America and the American Association of Health Plans, which have a history of supporting pediatric coverage expansions, could educate group health purchasers on the importance of accessible and affordable dependent coverage. These organizations could also illustrate to employers how improved coverage is in their economic interest.

Public health advocates could also educate Congress and state governments on the public health and economic benefits of providing public health insurance coverage for noncitizen children. States could increase their outreach activities to enroll eligible children in Medicaid or SCHIP programs and could use state funds to reach children whose coverage is not otherwise federally supported.

Finally, potential beneficiaries could be made aware of any improvements and expansions in eligibility for enrollment in Medicaid and/or SCHIP. Because of the complexity of enrollment, outreach activities that explain program benefits and provide help with enrollment are essential.

Funding Options. Both the federal and state governments would need to make additional funds available, through direct appropriations or tax incentives, to pay for these eligibility and coverage expansions. Congress could encourage increased state-level appropriations by conditioning the receipt of federal funding for *asthma-friendly* communities (see Recommendation 7.2) on state Medicaid and SCHIP expansions.

For employer-sponsored benefits, Congress could, through direct appropriations or the creation of tax incentives, make additional funds available to encourage employers to offer family coverage at subsidized rates. For recently arrived noncitizen children, Congress would need to pass new legislation to make all such children who meet other program requirements eligible for full Medicaid and SCHIP coverage.

Recommendation 5. Develop model benefit packages for essential childhood asthma services

Context. To reduce disparities in access to health care and in health outcomes, children with asthma must have insurance benefit packages commensurate with the appropriate standard of childhood asthma care. Otherwise, the actual level of care will be insufficient for all but the wealthiest children, whose families can afford to significantly supplement insurance coverage with out-of-pocket expenditures. Providing appropriate levels of health coverage to children with chronic conditions, including asthma, has been shown to significantly decrease hospital admissions and length of stay.[72]

Nevertheless, many medications and services essential to the proper treatment of children with persistent asthma, such as education in asthma self-management skills (see Recommendation 2) and case-management services (see Recommendation 3), may not be routinely covered by many private health insurance plans, who are unlikely to cover these services unless purchasers explicitly include them in their financial contracts with plans. These services also may not necessarily be covered by SCHIP programs, which are administered separately from Medicaid.

5.0 The Committee recommends that:

The appropriate agencies within the Department of Health and Human Services (Health Care Financing Administration, Centers for Disease Control and Prevention, and Health Resources and Services Administration), in collaboration with asthma-related professional and lay organizations, design a model insurance benefit package for children with asthma, based on the performance measures outlined in Recommendations 1–3. Specifically, the Committee recommends that:

5.1 Basic covered benefits for all children with asthma should be based on the National Asthma Education and Prevention Program (NAEPP) guidelines and include age-appropriate preventive medications and delivery devices, initial evaluation, self-management

education, and regular periodic management and follow-up (see Recommendations 1–2).

5.2 Basic benefits include referral to an asthma specialist under the conditions specified in the American Academy of Allergy, Asthma and Immunology taskforce guidelines.[36]

5.3 Extended benefits for children with moderate and severe persistent asthma include the case-management services described in Recommendation 3, as well as medically necessary durable medical equipment and supplies included in the NAEPP recommendations, such as nebulizers, spirometry, meters, and mattress covers.

5.4 The Department of Health and Human Services work with health care purchasing experts to translate model asthma-benefit packages into specific language that can be readily used by public and private health insurers to change and improve asthma benefits during contract negotiations with health plans. If certain extended benefits are deemed to fall beyond the limits of insurance, these services and interventions could be covered through public health grants (see Recommendation 7).

5.5 Since covered services under Medicaid are broadly defined and often subject to interpretation, it is particularly important that the Health Care Financing Administration make explicit those model asthma benefits (see 5.1, 5.2, and 5.3 above) that are currently covered by Medicaid, and that state Medicaid directors make sure that all contracting Medicaid providers cover these services (see Recommendation 6).

Implementation Options. The NAEPP would work with appropriate agencies in DHHS (CDC, HCFA, HRSA) to design a model benefit package for asthma, with accompanying documentation of the evidence base used to design the benefits. An organization with appropriate expertise would translate the model benefit package into contractual language so that health insurers could use this language in their negotiations with health plans. This process would be repeated periodically to ensure that benefits keep up with the latest clinical evidence. The goal would be to delineate important services, making sure government purchasers expect adherence to those services, and encouraging the private sector to do the same.

DHHS would also determine those model benefits that are not adopted by the private insurance market and target them in public health grant programs. The National Association of State Medicaid Directors' Maternal and Child Health Technical Advisory Group could also be instrumental in defining and implementing evidence-based insurance benefit packages for children with asthma on Medicaid. Public and private insurers could also augment their efforts to educate patients and providers regarding their benefits coverage. This would reduce possible misperceptions regarding the medications and services that are actually covered.

Funding Options. Funding for the development of asthma-specific contractual language for health care purchasers could come from a combination of public and private sources, including the Centers for Disease Control and Prevention, Health Resources and Services Administration, Medicaid, and health insurance associations (for example, the American Association of Health Plans and the Health Insurance Association of America). Asthma-related health insurance benefits would be funded through premium payments and Medicaid (see Recommendation 4). For uninsured children, these asthma-related services would be funded through the public health infrastructure (see Recommendation 7).

Recommendation 6. Educate health care purchasers about asthma benefits

Context. In the current climate of competition among managed care organizations, health care purchasers can use their market power to affect health care delivery patterns.[73] They have the opportunity, through the contracting process, to change benefits or to incorporate performance measures or guarantees. Thus, once model benefits packages are translated into asthma-specific contractual language (see Recommendation 5.4), it is important that this language be used by health care purchasers to negotiate contracts with health plans that incorporate evidence-based asthma benefits. To facilitate this process, purchasers of care could receive education and training on how to negotiate for high-quality asthma services, as well as accountability for those services. This education would stress the cost-effectiveness of quality childhood asthma care services.[55, 72]

6.0 The Committee recommends that:

Public and private health care purchasers, including large employers and Medicaid, be educated about how to negotiate contracts with health plans that include evidence-based asthma benefits (see Recommendation 5) and about accountability mechanisms that encourage the provision of quality asthma care. Specifically, the Committee recommends that:

6.1 Experts on asthma and on legal and financial contracts jointly conduct training courses for health care purchasers and provide purchasers with asthma-specific benefits language for inclusion in contractual agreements with health plans.

6.2 Purchasers be provided with and trained to use standardized, evidence-based performance measures (see Recommendations 1–3) that they can use to hold plans financially accountable for their performance.

Implementation Options. The education and training of health care purchasers could be facilitated by professional and private philanthropic organizations, such as the Robert Wood Johnson Foundation's Health Care Purchasing Institute. Such organizations have already developed some model programs for training and educating health care purchasers on how to use purchasing tools that translate standards of care into benefits language for inclusion in contractual agreements with health plans. The National Association of State Medicaid Directors' Maternal and Child Health Technical Advisory Group could play an instrumental role in educating and training state Medicaid program officers. Health care purchasing coalitions that have experience incorporating quality guidelines into contractual agreements, such as the Pacific Business Group on Health, could also play an important role.

Funding Options. Funds could be provided by the philanthropic organizations that support purchaser education. Health insurance organizations and employers may also wish to pay for the educational and technical assistance they receive, since it will benefit them financially in the long run.

Map of Health Care Delivery and Financing Policy Recommendations

Table 1 summarizes the recommendations for health care delivery and financing in relation to policy goals, funding options, and intervention sectors. A quick glance down a column reveals the comprehensiveness or specificity of a recommendation.

Table 1

Map of Health Care Delivery and Financing Policy Recommendations

	Policy Recommendations					
	Quality of Care Performance Measures			Coverage and Benefit Design		
	1	2	3	4	5	6
Related policy goals						
Improve health care	✔	✔	✔	✔	✔	✔
Improve asthma awareness	✔	✔	✔	✔	✔	✔
Ensure *asthma-friendly* schools		✔	✔		✔	
Promote *asthma-safe* home environments			✔		✔	
Reduce disparities	✔	✔	✔	✔	✔	✔
Promote innovation	✔		✔			✔
Funding options						
Public (federal/state/local)						✔
Both public and private	✔	✔	✔	✔	✔	✔
Intervention sector(s)						
Health care system	✔	✔	✔	✔	✔	✔
Education system		✔	✔			
Social services			✔		✔	
Environmental			✔		✔	

NOTE:

1 = Develop and implement primary care performance measures for childhood asthma care.

2 = Teach all children with persistent asthma and their families a specific set of self-management skills.

3 = Provide case-management to high-risk children.

4 = Extend continuous health insurance coverage to all uninsured children.

5 = Develop model benefit packages for essential childhood asthma services.

6 = Educate health care purchasers about asthma benefits.

STRENGTHENING THE PUBLIC HEALTH INFRASTRUCTURE

These recommendations are directed at the government agencies responsible for administering and funding public health functions that both support and supplement the health care delivery system. The recommendations fall into three subcategories: "Publicly Funding Asthma-Related Services That Fall Outside the Health Insurance System," "Increasing Public Awareness and Knowledge of Asthma," and "Improving Surveillance and Prevention Research Efforts."

Publicly Funding Asthma-Related Services That Fall Outside the Health Insurance System

The five recommendations in this category pertain to those personal and environmental health services that are essential to improving asthma outcomes but that are not feasibly financed through third-party insurance, either because they are not considered insurable services or because they are for individuals with no insurance coverage. These services include, for example, environmental health interventions that control exposure to asthma-provoking agents, and asthma prevention and management programs in schools.

Recommendation 7. Establish public health grants to foster *asthma-friendly* communities and home environments

Context. Focusing efforts solely on the traditional medical care and health insurance sectors will not adequately address the public health crisis represented by childhood asthma. A public health approach aimed at making communities *asthma-friendly* is needed to improve the health care of children with asthma and provide them with *asthma-safe* home environments

This type of public health approach has been used traditionally in the area of communicable diseases, such as tuberculosis and sexually transmitted disease. Asthma is similar in scope to these diseases, since it is affected by factors flowing from several health-related policy sectors (housing, education, workplace). Specifically, scientific evidence suggests that controlling certain elements of the indoor environment to which allergen-sensitive children with asthma are exposed (dust mites, fungi, cat hair, second-hand smoke) is an essential component of asthma control.[14] However, since allergen-reduction measures are only effective for those children who are allergen-sensitive, it is not yet clear if widespread allergen reduction is cost-effective. Research in this area should continue (see Recommendation 11).

The Children's Health Act of 2000 (see the Appendix) represents an important step toward expanding support for community-wide asthma prevention and management activities. The legislation, enacted by the 106th Congress in fall 2000, establishes asthma as a specific focus within the Public Health Service Act and authorizes appropriation of funds to improve the availability of treatment and prevention in communities with a high asthma prevalence, to upgrade asthma surveillance, and to support an interdisciplinary, cross-agency study of the federal role in asthma prevention. Thus, the legislation lays the groundwork for the development of a comprehensive national public policy in the area of asthma. If adequately supported through the congressional appropriations process, the legislation could, over time, provide communities facing a significant asthma problem with much-needed funds to improve services and coordinate activities.

7.0 The Committee recommends that:

Congress and the Department of Health and Human Services (DHHS) work together to ensure that the funding and implementation of the Children's Health Act of 2000 are adequate to provide essential childhood asthma services to children who fall outside of the health insurance system, and to promote *asthma-friendly* communities by addressing key environmental risk factors. Specifically, the Committee recommends that:

7.1 Over time, funding levels be increased to adequately support, at a minimum, the activities enumerated under the Act in all communities with high asthma prevalence, as defined by the Secretary of DHHS in accordance with the requirements of the new legislation and in consultation with experts. The following activities would be authorized as part of the Act's community grant program:

7.1.1 Provision of medically necessary durable medical equipment and supplies, (see Recommendation 5.3), at reduced or no cost to allergen-sensitive children with asthma whose insurance does not cover these services.

7.1.2 Provision of medical care, self-management education, and targeted case-management (see Recommendations 1–3) to children with persistent asthma who have no access to health insurance.

7.2 The Secretary consider establishing funding criteria that give states incentives to adopt additional policy reforms that would make new, federally funded activities more feasible and effective. Under this approach, the Secretary would make higher grant awards to states that adopt policies designed to address certain environmental risk factors for asthma. Incentives could include, but would not necessarily be limited to, the following:

7.2.1 Incentive payments to states that designate smoke-free areas in all congregate housing structures in which housing units are in sufficient proximity to cause exposure of nonsmoking residents.

7.2.2 Incentive payments to states that ensure that all Laundromats have specially designated washers that heat water to at least 130 degrees Fahrenheit, to eradicate mites from bedding.

7.2.3 Incentive payments to states that ensure that all schools in high-risk communities have a nurse or a designate who is trained in asthma management and education (see Recommendation 8.2).

7.3 Congress supplement the funds available under the Children's Health Act of 2000 to expand the Medicaid disproportionate-share hospital payment program to include additional funds that states can use for ambulatory and school health services located in and serving medically underserved communities. States' receipt of these funds would be contingent upon their use of a portion of the funds for the activities outlined in Recommendation 7.1.

Implementation Options. The strategies proposed here for implementing the Children's Health Act of 2000 would be formalized in consultation with representatives from state and local housing authorities, state and local school boards, small-business regulatory agencies, patient advocacy groups, the Department of Housing and Urban Development (HUD), the Environmental Protection Agency, and DHHS. In particular, HUD has two programs that can serve as models of successful collaboration between health and housing agencies to address housing-related health hazards: the Healthy Homes Initiative (HHI), which has addressed allergen control, and the Lead Hazard Control programs, which have distributed $552 million in lead-hazard-control grant funds to 112 grantees (local and state agencies) (personal communication with David J. Jacobs of the U.S. Department of Housing and Urban Development on December 8, 2000).

Funding Options. Funding for *asthma-friendly* communities would come from congressional appropriations for the newly authorized Children's Health Act of 2000 and from disproportionate-share funds for ambulatory care organizations (see Recommendation 7.3). Additional funds could come through appropriations for targeted programs such as HUD's HHI (see above), as well as tobacco tax revenues. Case-management services for children are covered for children who are on Medicaid. It is particularly important that Congress appropriate sufficient funds for the implementation of those asthma-related and other provisions of the Act that are not covered by Medicaid (see the Appendix).

Recommendation 8. Promote *asthma-friendly* schools and school-based asthma programs

Context. Asthma is a leading chronic illness–related cause of school absenteeism in the United States.[74] This problem is compounded by schools' concerns about their capacity to treat and manage these children while they are in school.[75, 76] Asthma-related absenteeism negatively affects both children's learning potential and parents' work productivity.[76, 77]

Examples of possible school-based programs include school-based asthma education,[78-81] school-based management of children with chronic asthma,[82] and assessment and control of environmental asthma triggers in schools (e.g. dusts, molds, and fungi). The EPA's *Indoor Air Quality Tools for Schools,*[31] which offers voluntary guidance to schools to assist them in developing indoor air quality management programs, is a promising approach that should be evaluated (see Recommendation 11).

Furthermore, the legal implications of school-based programs are important to consider. Children have rights under federal laws that prevent discrimination against individuals with disabilities (for example, the Americans with Disabilities Act and section 504 of the Rehabilitation Act) and under federal special-education law (the Individuals with Disabilities Education Act). These laws require schools to adopt reasonable modifications of the educational environment so that children with asthma receive an appropriate education.

The issue of schools' responsibility for children with asthma extends beyond federal education and disability law. Schools assume legal responsibility for the safety of children in their care during school hours. As a result, schools must be able to provide a safe environment for children. This duty is recognized not only in state education and civil tort laws but also in state nurse-practice acts, which require that schools have either their own nurse or someone supervised by a nurse, and which define specific nursing functions. For example, Maryland School health law mandates the use of school health services professionals, and the Maryland Nurse Practice Act mandates the training and supervision of school health assistants by nurses.[83, 84] These laws have helped expand school nursing services across the state.

8.0 The Committee recommends that:

The Department of Health and Human Services (DHHS) and the Department of Education, in collaboration with national state and local asthma organizations and local school boards, ensure that children with asthma benefit from comprehensive and coordinated school health programs nationwide. Specifically, the Committee recommends that:

8.1 State and local agencies establish performance measures for comprehensive asthma school services, based on the recommendations of the National Asthma Education and Prevention Program (NAEPP). These measures would cover access to a local or school-based clinic; assessment and initial treatment of acute symptoms that occur at school; adequate and immediate access to medications and delivery mechanisms during school hours; self-management education tailored to the school environment; linkages with case-management services; and encouragement of participation in sports and physical education.

8.2 School-based asthma services be physician or nurse-directed: Every school would have either a nurse or a designated health worker trained and supervised by a nurse, who is responsible for carrying out the asthma-related activities outlined in Recommendation 8.1.

8.3 Teachers with children with asthma in their classrooms receive in-service training on what to do in case of an acute asthma attack. Schools would develop and implement policies for classroom management of acute asthma cases.

8.4 National school professional and lay organizations educate school administrators and boards of education about the school-nurse laws in their states; the potential liability, under state and local laws, for lack of school asthma services; the revenue losses associated with asthma school absences; and examples of successful models for asthma school policies and practices.

Implementation Options. The appropriate agencies in DHHS, the Department of Education, and the School Subcommittee of NAEPP would develop performance measures and coordinate national-level dissemination and education activities with direct involvement and participation of states and the American Association of Health Plans, many of whose member plans are involved in the provision of school-site care. For example, the Health Resources and Services Administration, which oversees health professions' education and training programs for the federal government, could develop school-nurse education programs designed to upgrade school nurses' asthma management skills. The appropriate health and professional groups (National Association of State Boards of Education, National Association of School Nurses, National Association of School Administrators, American School Health Association, American Public Health Association Section of School Nurses, and American Academy of Pediatrics) would also be involved in disseminating and implementing national performance measures.

The National Education Association and community-based advocacy organizations would educate parents on how to advocate for school health services to which children with asthma are entitled under the law. These organizations would also educate school officials on the legal requirements in their states and identify model school asthma programs that comply with those requirements.

The Department of Education under the Clinton administration supported a bipartisan bill in Congress to fund the building and modernization of schools to, among other things, provide *asthma-friendly* indoor environments. Similar bills should continue to be supported and passed. In addition, children with asthma may be eligible to receive special education and related services under the Individuals with Disabilities Education Act. Benefits under this Act could be explored at the state and local levels in an effort to integrate health and education services for school children with asthma.

Funding Options. Congress could make funds available to DHHS and the Department of Education for asthma-related school health services and education activities. While the Children's Health Act of 2000 does not specifically mention school-based asthma services, there is nothing to prevent activities authorized under the Act from taking place in schools. Thus, schools could be promoted as an appropriate venue for the services covered by the Act.

Medicaid covers certain health services furnished by nurses and other licensed health professionals in schools that comply with Medicaid participation requirements. Schools should be made aware of and take full advantage of these Medicaid-reimbursable services. In addition, Congress could revise the Medicaid program, as described in Recommendation 7.3, to furnish additional direct Medicaid funding through the disproportionate-share payment program to school-based programs that disproportionately serve children on Medicaid or State Children's Health Insurance Program programs.

Ideally, school-based services would be covered as a community benefit rather than an insurance benefit. Such a community benefit would be available to all children who attend school (regardless of their Medicaid status), with financing through local and other special taxes, such as health insurance premium taxes, ensuring that health insurers who derive the financial benefits of better ongoing asthma management help support such programs. These sources of revenues could be supplemented by federal funds, such as funds furnished through the Title V Maternal and Child Health Services Block Grant, the Prevention Block Grant, Federal School Health funding, and funds appropriated under the Children's Health Act of 2000.

Increasing Public Awareness and Knowledge of Asthma

This recommendation addresses the need for broad public education aimed at improving public awareness and support of asthma treatment and prevention efforts.

Recommendation 9. Launch a national asthma public education campaign

Context. Despite recent alarming increases in the prevalence and incidence of asthma,[1, 2, 85] evidence indicates that ignorance about asthma risk factors, symptoms, and management is widespread.[86] Increasing public awareness of asthma will not only reinforce patient-focused educational efforts (see Recommendation 2) but will also help friends and family to identify children with asthma who are not currently getting appropriate medical attention. It is especially important that national educational messages be adapted to the cultural and linguistic needs of local communities.

Lessons on how to launch a successful national asthma media campaign can be learned from Australia's experience.[87] The Australian campaign targeted people with undiagnosed and underdiagnosed asthma. The goal was to encourage these people to seek medical attention and learn new ways of preventing asthma exacerbations, thereby promoting a symptom-free life. The campaign applied social marketing principles and used focus groups to develop the media messages. Television was the principal medium chosen, and a famous sports figure was used as a spokesperson. An evaluation of the campaign showed a significant increase in asthma awareness and knowledge among the public, as well as improvements in self-reported asthma management among patients with asthma.[87] Decreased hospital readmission rates among patients with asthma have also been documented, although such declines are likely the result of improvements in care.[88]

9.0 The Committee recommends that:

The Department of Health and Human Services (DHHS), in collaboration with the National Asthma Education and Prevention Program (NAEPP), national professional organizations, and state and private agencies, develop and implement a national asthma public education campaign that expands on current efforts. Specifically, the Committee recommends that:

9.1 The asthma public education campaign be designed to increase community-wide awareness of the prevalence and severity of the disease, as well as to increase symptom recognition among children with asthma and their families.

9.2 The Surgeon General be the principal spokesperson for the campaign, and bring together public and private organizations, including sports organizations, to develop and deliver media messages targeted to specific populations.

9.3 National asthma organizations provide technical assistance to community-based efforts to promote asthma awareness.

Implementation Options. To implement this recommendation, the Patient and Public Education Subcommittee of the NAEPP could expand its current media-related public education efforts. Through its membership in the NAEPP, the Environmental Protection Agency is working with the Ad Council to raise public awareness about asthma, focusing on controlling environmental triggers as part of a comprehensive asthma management plan. This multimedia advertising campaign is targeting African Americans, Hispanics, and low-income, urban residents. As part of this campaign, Allergy and Asthma Network/Mothers of Asthmatics, Inc., will staff an asthma hotline that will be available to the general public to call for additional asthma information. To expand the scope of this message and of the target group, the NAEPP could bring together media experts (including the Ad Council), pharmaceutical companies, asthma experts, and the Asthma and Allergy Foundation of America and the American Lung Association to devise a strategy for a national media campaign. Although it is difficult to attribute changes in knowledge, attitudes, and behaviors to such a campaign, an evaluative component could be part of the campaign. To foster national-local interactions, national asthma-related organizations (for example, the NAEPP, Centers for Disease Control and Prevention, ALA) could provide technical assistance to local organizations and promote the creation of community-based coalitions to coordinate local community educational campaigns.

Funding Options. The national asthma media campaign could be funded in part through congressional appropriations to DHHS. Philanthropic organizations could provide funds to support formation of a coalition to design the message and identify the target group. Pharmaceutical companies could be approached for additional funding, and network broadcasting companies could be asked to donate airtime.

Improving Surveillance and Prevention Research Efforts

The two recommendations in this area are for improving the research evidence on which primary and secondary preventive interventions are based and for improving the population-based tracking mechanisms that help direct asthma health care resources in the most appropriate manner.

Recommendation 10. Develop a national asthma surveillance system

Context: An essential tool for promoting access to quality asthma care and improving the health of children with asthma is an asthma surveillance system that can capture condition-specific information at the national, state, and community levels. A good surveillance system will provide an accurate assessment of the magnitude and nature of the childhood asthma crisis and will help guide appropriate allocation of resources to address it effectively.

The nation's current asthma monitoring capacity is very limited compared with existing infrastructures for other important health concerns, such as tuberculosis, sexually transmitted diseases, and immunizations. This limitation is largely due to the complexity of asthma diagnosis, which requires a combination of symptoms, measurement of lung function, and observation over time. The only asthma-specific data currently available at the state, county, city, and census-tract levels are mortality data,[2] which are inadequate for developing strategies for prevention, treatment, and management, because they tell health authorities who has asthma only when it is too late. National data on asthma prevalence, hospitalizations, outpatient visits, and emergency department visits are reported at the regional level only and thus do not allow for the planning of city- or state-specific evaluations and interventions. In addition, these data are not available until several years after collection. An evaluation of states' capacities to conduct asthma surveillance showed that limited availability of reliable data at the local level and a lack of administrative infrastructure greatly hampered states' efforts.[89] As of 1998, fewer than 10 states had conducted asthma prevalence surveys.[85]

In response to the need for improved asthma surveillance, the Centers for Disease Control and Prevention, with National Institutes of Health and Environmental Protection Agency funds, have begun to develop national standards for asthma surveillance and models for state and local asthma surveillance, using existing data. These efforts mark important first steps. However, a more coordinated and better-funded effort will be necessary to create a national system that captures reliable real-time data on prevalence, incidence, and severity of asthma, as well as information about the quality of asthma management.

10.0 The Committee recommends that:

The federal government spearhead the creation of a national population-based asthma surveillance system with participation from state and local governments. Specifically, the Committee recommends that:

10.1 The Centers for Disease Control and Prevention (CDC), in collaboration with state agencies, providers, and payers, establish and refine national standards for asthma surveillance, including the content of information to be collected, the merging of data from different sources, and reporting requirements. The surveillance measures chosen would make it possible to chart progress toward the asthma-related *Healthy People 2010* objectives.

10.2 Congress and state legislatures provide matching funds to create and operate state and local asthma surveillance units to carry out these standard-driven activities, including more-detailed assessment of risk factors in communities with outcomes worse than average.

10.3 The CDC work with states to identify appropriate sentinel events for asthma, such as admission to an intensive care unit, intubation, need for resuscitation measures, or death. Once identified, such events would be reported and would require strategic action plans for appropriate medical follow-up.

Implementation Options. The CDC would lead the effort to establish surveillance standards and would work with other federal agencies and state health departments to ensure the appropriateness of the standards. The National Center for Health Statistics could work with asthma experts to use the asthma-related data from current national surveys (such as the National Health Interview Survey, the National Health and Nutrition Examination Survey, the National Hospital Discharge Survey, the National Ambulatory Medical Care Survey, and the National Vital Statistics System). The CDC could also use Health Care Financing Administration (HCFA) Medicaid data on eligibility, claims, and expenditures to compare asthma-related costs over time for continuously enrolled children versus those for intermittent or short-time enrollees. Specifically, the (HCFA Office of Strategic Planning, Research and Evaluation Group, Division of Beneficiary Studies, conducts research on asthma, much of which focuses on prevention and potentially preventable high-cost care (from personal communication with M. Beth Benedict of HCFA on December 6, 2000). Finally, many health plans have developed their own performance measures to track asthma outcomes for their enrollees. The American Association of Health Plans could be involved in linking these plan-level data systems to a national surveillance system.

Once the CDC and the Council of State and Territorial Epidemiologists, in consultation with the American College of Emergency Physicians, American Academy of Family Physicians, and the American Academy of Pediatrics, and other professional organizations, agree on an appropriate notifiable asthma-related event, health care providers and state health departments would work together on implementing a reporting mechanism that includes a system for appropriate medical follow-up. Such a system could be modeled on the CDC's current fetal and infant mortality notification process. The burden and potential liability associated with knowing about a near-death episode and not being able to respond is a potential barrier that should be considered by legal experts. However, the potential for intervening on behalf of a fairly small population in need of medical attention makes the reporting of near-death events an important goal of a good asthma notification system.

Funding Options. Funding for a national asthma surveillance system would be allocated by Congress. Provisions for such funding are included in Subtitle D of the Children's Health Act of 2000 (see the Appendix). States and local communities could also provide funding, possibly assisted by matching funds from federal and state sources, respectively.

Recommendation 11. Develop and implement a national agenda for asthma prevention research

Context. Recent dramatic increases in asthma prevalence and the continuing burden of the disease present a special challenge to asthma researchers. Important primary and secondary asthma prevention research to date has laid the groundwork for additional clinical, epidemiological, behavioral, and health services research in this area. Basic science research should continue at its current pace. But a significant funding boost for asthma research in humans in their natural settings is necessary to investigate and identify the possible environmental, genetic, and lifestyle factors associated with asthma prevalence and morbidity. More research is necessary on health care system factors and their role in improving asthma management, such as the effectiveness of quality improvement strategies in different patient populations and circumstances. This knowledge from applied and clinical research will allow development of effective environmental and health care system primary and secondary prevention interventions.

Basic research on the etiology of asthma should continue to be a key part of a national agenda for primary prevention research. However, key sociodemographic and environmental risk factors for childhood asthma, including allergen exposure, second-hand smoke, socio-economic status, and obesity,[14, 90-95] have already been associated with asthma prevalence and the worsening of symptoms in people with the illness. Until the underlying causes of the increase in asthma prevalence are better understood, secondary prevention research should focus on these known risk factors and on strategies to increase adherence (health professional and patient) to effective asthma management practices. Regions and subpopulations at highest risk should be targeted for this research.

Various research funding agencies within the Department of Health and Human Services (DHHS) have already identified asthma as a priority area, so the next step in advancing asthma primary and secondary prevention research must involve formal articulation of the research agenda and coordination of funding streams.

11.0 The Committee recommends that:

The Department of Health and Human Services, in collaboration with other federal and state health and environmental agencies, develop and implement a national agenda for research on primary and secondary asthma prevention, with an augmentation of funding for the epidemiologic, clinical, and behavioral sciences. Specifically, the Committee recommends that:

11.1 Basic science and epidemiological primary prevention research focus on the causes and natural history of asthma, including the causes of the recent increase in the prevalence and severity of asthma, and variations in the spectrum of the disease.

11.2 Secondary prevention research focus on the causes of asthma exacerbations and strategies to prevent them, and on identifying the barriers to adequate management of the disease and interventions to overcome those barriers. Intervention aimed at controlling indoor environmental triggers, especially in schools, would also be rigorously evaluated.

11.3 Prevention researchers elucidate the reasons for disparities in asthma-related outcomes among subgroups of the population and work toward eliminating those disparities. Studies in this area would examine the role of the physical environment, lifestyle, gene-environment interactions, and health care interventions, such as case-management. Community-based interventions would be evaluated in the populations experiencing the greatest burden of disease.

11.4 Prevention researchers work to develop improved measurement tools for conducting population-based surveillance (see Recommendation 10.1) and monitoring the quality of asthma care (see Recommendation 1.2), to achieve the goals outlined in Recommendations 1 and 10. In addition, current data sources would be refined and new sources explored, so that surveillance and performance measures can be captured in a reliable and valid manner.

Implementation Options. The details of the prevention research agenda would be developed by the Department of Health and

Human Services, in collaboration with the National Asthma Education and Prevention Program and relevant philanthropic organizations. Active and prominent interdisciplinary asthma researchers will consult in this process. The federal agencies that would be involved include the following:

- National Heart, Lung, and Blood Institute
- National Institute of Allergy and Infectious Diseases
- Agency for Healthcare Research and Quality
- Centers for Disease Control and Prevention
- Environmental Protection Agency
- Health Care Financing Administration
- National Institute of Child Health and Human Development
- National Institutes of Nursing Research
- National Institute of Environmental Health Sciences.

The collaborative and diverse research agenda will provide guidance to individual agencies as they determine their own specific research plans that fulfill their respective agency mission.

Funding Options. The national asthma prevention research agenda would be funded through congressional appropriations to DHHS, the National Institutes of Health, the Agency for Healthcare Research and Quality, and other federal research agencies. Additional unrestricted funds for research could be solicited from the pharmaceutical industry and from other private organizations. Private organizations' investments in research would promote the public good and may result in other long-term benefits.

Map of Public Health Infrastructure Policy Recommendations

Table 2 summarizes the recommendations for strengthening the public health infrastructure, in relation to policy goals, funding options, and intervention sectors. A quick glance down a column reveals the comprehensiveness or specificity of a recommendation.

Table 2

Map of Public Health Infrastructure Policy Recommendations

	Policy Recommendation				
	Uninsured Community and Health Services		Public Aware-ness	Surveillance and Research	
	7	8	9	10	11
Related policy goals					
Improve health care	✔	✔		✔	✔
Improve asthma awareness	✔	✔	✔	✔	✔
Ensure *asthma-friendly* schools	✔	✔	✔		✔
Promote *asthma-safe* home environments	✔		✔	✔	✔
Reduce disparities	✔	✔	✔	✔	✔
Promote innovation	✔	✔		✔	✔
Funding options					
Public (federal/state/local)	✔			✔	✔
Both public and private		✔	✔		
Intervention sector(s)					
Health care system	✔	✔	✔	✔	✔
Education system	✔	✔	✔	✔	✔
Social services	✔	✔	✔		✔
Environmental	✔	✔	✔	✔	✔

NOTE:

7 = Establish public health grants to foster *asthma-friendly* communities and home environments.

8 = Promote *asthma-friendly* schools and school-based asthma programs.

9 = Launch a national asthma public education campaign.

10 = Develop a national asthma surveillance system.

11 = Develop and implement a national agenda for asthma prevention research.

Chapter Six

CONCLUSION

If fully implemented, the recommendations described in this report would lead to major improvements in childhood asthma outcomes in the United States and would increase the number of *asthma-friendly* communities. These recommendations, which focus on prevention, treatment, and management of asthma and on the integration of community asthma prevention activities, are strongly related. At the same time, as with many public policy recommendations, they could be adopted in stages and over time.

The timing of this report in tandem with the passage of the "Asthma Services for Children" title of the Children's Health Act of 2000 is quite fortunate. The congressional attention provided by this Act builds on multiple public and private childhood asthma efforts to date and creates additional momentum for implementing the kind of national childhood policy agenda outlined in this report.

NEXT STEPS

The recommendations in this report encompass a range of public and private strategies and provide a blueprint for developing new and existing national childhood asthma activities and for coordinating those activities. This blueprint is intended to shape discussions among the key stakeholders and actors who must further develop the policy options described here. We hope this document will be a working guide for coordinating the activities of both public and private organizations at the federal, state, and local community level. We would like the blueprint to provide inspiration for innovative ways to strengthen the collaboration and communication among national and local community leaders and programs in order to successfully translate these national policies into local community practices.

We envision several possible next steps for this effort. Given the central role of the National Asthma Education and Prevention Program (NAEPP) in our recommendations, we would call for additional funding and resources to expand its current activities. The membership of the NAEPP and its working committees provide an appropriate organizational structure for coordinating the policies outlined in this report. No other organization in the United States today broadly represents the multiple perspectives that are necessary to address the national problem of childhood asthma. The creation of a new NAEPP Health Care Policy and Financing Subcommittee, including current and new members who are key stakeholders, would facilitate the initial discussion of the recommendations and the process of further development and implementation.

In addition, or in collaboration with NAEPP efforts, public and private funders could also support a series of national meetings or workshops to formulate more specific policy actions and implementation strategies according to the areas described in this blueprint. Working groups corresponding to the policy categories or the subcategories described in this report could be formed to provide a forum for identifying omissions in content and alternative viewpoints. These working groups could include the major funding and legal authorities responsible for implementing the proposed policies. For instance, meetings with Medicaid and state policymakers would serve to communicate the urgency of dealing with asthma and delineate strategies to ascertain potential impact of interventions, such as case-management, that Medicaid and the State Children's Health Insurance Program can pay for.

Because the recommendations are interrelated and because all are necessary for implementing a comprehensive national agenda, it would probably be helpful to repeat a structured panel meeting like the one described in this report. A future iteration would focus on explicit coordination of existing and new programs and agencies and identify concrete plans for interagency collaborations, specifying timelines, appropriations levels, and responsible parties. The Children's Health Act of 2000 (Title V, Subtitle C) calls for such a coordination of federal asthma activities (see the Appendix), which would provide a natural forum for considering the policy recommendations in this report.

IMPLICATIONS OF THE CHILDREN'S HEALTH ACT OF 2000

In a number of instances, the Children's Health Act of 2000 may permit the types of improvements contained in the policy recommendations of this report. Indeed, if appropriately funded, the Act could provide much-needed support at the national and local levels for improvements in access to asthma prevention and management services.

By identifying asthma as a national health priority for the first time, the Act represents an important step in national asthma policy. It recognizes the importance of creating a national asthma policy and provides aid to local, particularly hard-hit, communities.

At the same time, it is important to note the limitations of the Act.

First, whether the Act will be adequately funded remains to be seen. Before the Act can take effect, as with all discretionary programs, requires that Congress enact accompanying spending legislation as part of the Labor/Health and Human Services appropriations process.

Second, the Act does not make changes in public and private insurance programs. Although designed to address some of the community public health issues raised in this report, the Act is not designed to address deficiencies in insurance coverage. Nor does the Act authorize the Secretary to condition state awards on the adoption of comprehensive insurance reforms (although, as discussed earlier, the adoption of performance incentives would seem permissible). These reforms await separate congressional and state legislative action.

Finally, the Act does not address basic deficiencies in housing stock and housing infrastructure that exacerbate asthma. Although funds could be used to improve community living conditions, they are modest and would fall short of what is needed to upgrade housing.

FEDERAL LEGISLATION RELEVANT TO CHILDHOOD ASTHMA

INTRODUCTION

Legislation related to childhood asthma was introduced and considered during the 106th Congress. This Appendix reviews that legislation. After summarizing the methodology used to carry out this review, we analyze those measures related to the authorization of new childhood asthma-related activities on which both House and Senate legislative action were completed as of the end of September 2000.

This analysis indicates that childhood asthma–related public policy constituted a significant focus of federal legislative activities during the 106th Congress. The result of this focus is significant new legislative authority on health care–related matters generally, and in the areas of asthma prevention, treatment, management, and research specifically. Furthermore, although community prevention activities beyond those specifically connected to the provision of health care did not receive as much attention, the legislation authorizes an important new study that could result in a greater national understanding of the role that community living conditions and the quality of public housing play in preventing and reducing asthma.

METHODS AND RESULTS

We used standard legislative research techniques to prepare this analysis, beginning with a computerized search of "Thomas" (the congressional website) on September 13, 22, and 28, 2000. The purpose of the search was to identify any legislation that specifically incorporated the terms "asthma", "childhood asthma", or "asthma" and "children." The search process was repeated several times, because it is customary for legislation that is pending to move rapidly and change status in the final weeks of the federal fiscal year.

This search process yielded 32 separate pieces of legislation introduced during the 106th Congress and containing the term "asthma." Because "Thomas" is designed to reflect congressional proceedings for which each phase of the congressional deliberation process results in a separately identifiable reported bill, in a number of cases several entries actually pertained to the same measure at different stages of the legislative process.

From the 32 asthma entries, we were able to identify the following principal measures introduced during the process:

1. Asthma Act (H.R. 1965)
2. Children's Asthma Relief Act (H.R. 2840, S. 805)
3. Asthma Awareness, Education and Treatment Act of 1999 (H.R. 1966)
4. Urban Asthma Reduction Act of 1999 (H.R. 875)
5. Children's Health Research and Prevention Amendments of 1999 (H.R. 3301)
6. Children's Public Health Act of 2000 (S. 2868)
7. Children's Health Act of 2000 (H.R. 4365)
8. Asthma Inhalers Regulatory Relief Act of 1999 (H.R. 136)
9. National Latex Allergy Awareness Week (H. Con. Res. 387)
10. National Alpha 1 Awareness Month (S. Res. 84)
11. Native Hawaiian Health Care Improvement Act Reauthorization of 1999 (S. 1929); reported in the Senate (S. 1929)
12. Pregnancy Discrimination Act Amendments of 2000 (H.R. 3861)
13. Public Health Osteoporosis Screening, Diagnosis and Treatment Act of 1999 (H.R. 2471)

14. Safe Medications for the Elderly Act of 2000 (H.R. 5140)
15. Clean Power Plant Act of 1999 (H.R. 2980)
16. Clean Power Plant and Modernization Act of 1999 (S. 1949)
17. Grants to Improve the Infrastructure of Elementary and Secondary Schools (H.R. 3071; H.R. 1820)
18. School Environment Protection Act of 1999 (H.R. 3275; S. 2109)
19. Public School Modernization and Overcrowding Relief Act of 1999 (S. 1454)
20. School Environment Protection Act of 1999 (S. 1716)
21. Comprehensive Health Access District Act (H.R. 298; H.R. 304)
22. Children's Health Insurance Accountability Act of 1999 (S. 636; H.R. 1661)
23. Social Security and Medicare Safe Deposit Box Act of 2000 (H.R. 4577)
24. Departments of Labor, Health and Human Services and Education and Related Agencies Appropriations Act, 2001 (H.R. 4577)

After briefly examining each of these introduced measures, we determined that they pertained to many of the issues that ultimately were included in final legislation. They also are an indication of the extent to which policymakers are broadly aware of the dimensions of the asthma problem and interested in identifying public policy interventions.

The areas addressed by the legislation covered the following matters: the general problem of insurance coverage for children; funds to ensure greater protections against asthma and access to basic asthma management and prevention in schools and communities; expansion of community health services related to asthma; and public education related to childhood asthma.

Substandard housing was one significant problem that did not appear to receive specific legislative recognition. The absence of asthma-related public housing legislation suggests either that the problem of substandard housing and its impact on asthma is not fully understood or that there is at present insufficient legislative support, even on an initial basis, for legislation aimed specifically at asthma-related housing improvements.*

A review of the legislation also suggests that the most active members of Congress on asthma-specific matters are from urban areas, where the asthma problem may be greatest and easiest to recognize. Almost all bills were introduced by members of Congress who represent urban districts, and several of the most important measures received bipartisan support from the start. This bipartisan approach to children's health issues has been a hallmark of Congress for decades.**

The legislative history for the bills is as follows:

- Various measures were referred to the Committees of Jurisdiction in both Houses.
- A series of separate measures pertaining to both childhood asthma and other matters was combined and reported in the form of omnibus legislation to authorize new activities related to childhood asthma. This legislation (The Children's Health Act of 2000, H.R. 4365) passed the House of Representatives on May 9, 2000.
- The House bill was then *engrossed in* (sent to and received by) the Senate, where several amendments were added on the Senate floor. Floor action occurred in the Senate on September 22, 2000.
- On September 27, 2000, the House of Representatives took up the Senate-passed version of the legislation and voted (395 to 25) to approve the bill as amended and send it to the President, who signed it into law on October 17, 2000.

---

*This is not to suggest that there is not support for general improvements in public housing, only that the issue of housing reform tied specifically to asthma reduction did not appear in the legislation.

**Many of the most important measures to emerge around child-health improvement over the past 30 years have been strongly bipartisan. The most prominent examples of this bipartisanship in the area of children's health are the Medicaid reforms enacted between 1984 and 1990 and the creation of the State Children's Health Insurance Program (SCHIP).

A DESCRIPTION OF THE CHILDREN'S HEALTH ACT OF 2000

The Children's Health Act of 2000 is an omnibus piece of legislation that addresses numerous issues in child health. The asthma-related provisions of the Act consolidate a number of the smaller asthma-related measures introduced in the 106th Congress. The Act comprises 35 separate titles pertaining to children's health, as well as drug and mental-health services for youth.

Title V: Programs Related to Asthma

Title V of the Act (H.R. 4365, Title V), entitled "Asthma Services for Children," contains provisions of direct relevance to this analysis. It amends the Public Health Service Act (PHS Act) to create several new asthma-related program funding authorities.* In addition, Title V amends one existing PHS Act health program to strengthen its role in the prevention of asthma.

Title V contains four subtitles: "Asthma Services," "Prevention Activities," "Coordination of Federal Activities," and "Compilation of Data."

Subtitle A: Asthma Services. The Act amends Title III of the Public Health Service Act to expand and strengthen preventive, treatment, and health and health-related asthma management services. Funds are authorized for five years, a typical length of time for health service programs authorized under the Public Health Service Act.

Title V of the Act adds a new Part P (§399L.) authorizing and requiring the Secretary to make awards to "eligible entities." An *eligible entity* is a "public or private non-profit private entity (including a state or political subdivision of a state) or a consortium of any such entities. (§399L(a)(3)). The awards are for the following purposes:

- To provide "quality medical care" for children who live in "areas that have a high prevalence of asthma" and who "lack access to medical care" (§399L(a)(1)(A)).

---

*As of the end of September 2000, no final appropriations legislation for FY 2001 had been established. Therefore, it is not possible to report on the final funding levels for Title V.

- To provide "on-site education" to parents, children, health care providers, and "medical teams" to recognize the signs and symptoms of asthma, and to train them in the use of medications to treat asthma and "prevent its exacerbations [sic]" (§399L(a)(1)(B)).
- To decrease "preventable trips to the emergency room" by making "medication" available to "individuals who have not previously had access to treatment or education in the management of asthma" (§399L(a)(1)(C)).
- To provide other services, such as smoking-cessation programs, home modification, and other direct and support services that "ameliorate conditions that exacerbate or induce asthma" (§399L(a)(1)(D)).

In making grants, the authorizing language (§399L(a)(2)) specifies that the Secretary may, but is not required to,* make grants that develop and expand certain projects:

- Projects to provide "comprehensive asthma services to children" in accordance with National Asthma Education and Prevention Program guidelines, including access to "care and treatment for asthma in a community-based setting" (§399L(a)(2)(A)).
- Projects to "fully equip" mobile health care clinics that provide "preventive asthma care," including diagnosis, physical examinations, pharmacological therapy, skin testing, peak-flow-meter testing, and other asthma-related health care services" (§399L(a)(2)(B)).
- Projects to conduct "validated asthma management education programs" for patients with asthma and their families, including "patient education regarding asthma management, family education on asthma management, and the distribution of materials, including displays and videos, to reinforce concepts presented by medical teams" (§399L(a)(2)(C)).

---

*Specific appropriations language may, of course, limit the Secretary's discretion with respect to the funding of these authorized activities.

The Secretary may award grants under the law and must give preference to eligible entities that

> demonstrate that the activities to be carried out under this section shall be in localities within areas of known or suspected high prevalence of childhood asthma or high asthma-related mortality or high rate of hospitalization or emergency room visits for asthma (relative to the average asthma prevalence rates and associated mortality rates in the United States) (§399L(a)(2)(A)[sic]).

The Act specifies what can constitute "acceptable data sets" to include the following:

> Data from Federal, state or local vital statistics, claims data under title XIX [Medicaid] or XXI [State Children's Health Insurance Program (SCHIP)] of the Social Security Act, other public health statistics or surveys, claims data under title XIX or XXI of the Social Security Act, other public health statistics or surveys, or other data that the Secretary, in consultation with the Director of the Centers for Disease Control and Prevention deems appropriate (§399L(a)(2)(B) [sic]).

In their grant applications, eligible entities must identify how they will coordinate grant-supported activities with programs operated under Medicaid, SCHIP, the state Maternal and Child Health Services Block Grant, child welfare and foster care and adoption assistance programs, Head Start, WIC, local "public and private" elementary or secondary schools, or public housing agencies (§399L(b)).

Eligible entities that receive funding must provide evaluations of the operations and activities carried out under the grant. The evaluations must include a description of the health status outcomes of assisted children, an assessment of asthma-related health care utilization services, the collection, analysis, and reporting of data according to Centers for Disease Control and Prevention (CDC)-developed guidelines, and such other information as the Secretary may require (§399L(c)).

The level of authorized appropriations for the service program is "such sums as may be necessary" for fiscal years 2001–2005.*

Subtitle B: Prevention Activities. Subtitle B amends the Preventive Health and Health Services Block Grant (§1901 et seq. of the Public Health Service Act) to add a new category of authorized activities to establish, operate, and coordinate

> effective and cost-efficient systems to reduce the prevalence of illness due to asthma and asthma related illnesses, especially among children, by reducing the level of exposure to cockroach allergen or other known asthma triggers through the use of integrated pest management as applied to cockroaches or other known allergens (§1904(a)(1)(E), as added by Subtitle B, Title V).

Allowable expenditures under this new authority may include "the costs of building maintenance and the costs of programs to promote community participation in the carrying out of integrated pest management, as applied to cockroaches or other known allergens" (§1904(a)(1)(E), as added by Subtitle B, Title V).

No additional funding is authorized for this activity, since the Preventive Health Block Grant already is authorized on a "such sums" basis.**

Subtitle C: Coordination of Federal Asthma Activities. Subtitle C directs the Director of the National Heart, Lung and Blood Institute, through the National Asthma Education Prevention Program, to

- Identify all federal programs that carry out asthma-related activities
- Develop, "in consultation with appropriate federal agencies and professional and voluntary health organizations, a federal plan for responding to asthma"

---

*The determination of necessity under legislation such as this is made by Congress as part of the annual appropriations process. The legislation authorizes discretionary spending, rather than entitlement spending up to the level of need.

**Thus, the important question is whether FY 2001 appropriations levels for the Block Grant will be increased to reflect this new activity.

- Not later than 12 months after the date of enactment of the Children's Health Act, submit recommendations to the appropriate committees of Congress on ways to strengthen and improve the coordination of asthma-related activities of the federal government (§424B(a) of the Public Health Service Act, as added by Subtitle C, Title V).

The Director is required to include a representative from the United States Department of Housing and Urban Development in the NAEPP for the purpose of carrying out this federal study (§424B(a) of the Public Health Service Act, as added by Subtitle C, Title V). The legislation authorizes such sums as are necessary for carrying out the study.

Subtitle D: Compilation of Data. The Act amends the Public Health Service Act to require the Director of the CDC to conduct local surveillance activities to collect data on asthma prevalence and severity, and to compile and annually publish data on national childhood mortality related to asthma. The legislation authorizes such sums as may be necessary to carry out the activity.

CONCLUSION AND IMPLICATIONS

The Children's Health Act of 2000 contains important national public policy advances in childhood asthma prevention, treatment, management, and surveillance. The new grant-making authority under the law will provide funds to communities with a high prevalence of childhood asthma to improve the delivery and coordination of health. For communities with an elevated prevalence of asthma, it will provide funds for preventive education services. To the extent that state health agencies, consistent with the prevention provisions of the Act, redirect prevention health block grant funding and resources to pest-control activities, the legislation may yield increased investment in the control of known allergens. The identification of asthma as an area for the development of surveillance activities represents a statement of congressional concern regarding the importance of community health monitoring as part of an overall national policy strategy to reduce the impact and severity of asthma. Finally, the national policy study required under the Act will provide a framework for augmented activities that extend beyond the provision of health care and that reach critical issues related to the quality of housing and the community environment.

The Act is broad in scope and, if fully funded (that is, funded up to the level of defined need), could provide assistance to communities with high asthma prevalence. Inevitably, of course, actual funding may be below full need levels, as is the case with some PHS Act programs. Furthermore, the legislation does not contain improvements in insurance coverage for children, although legislation currently pending in Congress would, if enacted, increase the potential for coverage of particularly vulnerable groups of children, including recently arrived immigrant children. Nonetheless, the program represents movement toward a national asthma policy.

The success of the legislation will depend on more than funding levels. As drafted, the Act vests broad discretion in the Secretary of Health and Human Services to define key terms such as "high prevalence," "validated asthma management programs," "lack of access to management care," and other key terms that ultimately will determine who can qualify for funding and allowable uses of funds. In addition, the Secretary has discretion within the limits of the law (and such other limits that may be imposed as part of the appropriations process) to identify funding priorities, establish grant qualification standards, and determine what constitutes permissible expenditures and required inter-program coordination activities. How these decisions are made, the extent to which implementation includes consultation with experts in programs to which this new authority must relate, and the standards that emerge, will significantly further the ultimate reach of the program.

Finally, the legislation vests considerable discretion in states and communities to design interventions that meet local need. Evaluation of the program's components and states' responses to the legislation will be an important part of furthering the development of national asthma policy.

REFERENCES

1. U.S. Department of Health and Human Services, *Action Against Asthma: A Strategic Plan for the Department of Health and Human Services*, Washington, D.C., 2000.

2. Mannino, D. M., D. M. Homa, C. A. Pertowski, A. Ashizawa, et al., "Surveillance for Asthma—United States, 1960–1995," *Morbidity and Mortality Weekly Report (MMWR), CDC Surveillance Summaries*, Vol. 47, No. 1, pp. 1–27.

3. Adams, P. F., and M. A. Marano, "Current Estimates from the National Health Interview Survey, 1994," *Vital Health Statistics*, Vol. 1094, 1995.

4. Carter-Pokras, O. D., and P. J. Gergen, "Reported Asthma Among Puerto Rican, Mexican-American, and Cuban Children, 1982 through 1984," *American Journal of Public Health*, Vol. 83, No. 4, 1993, pp. 580–582.

5. Halfon, N., and P. W. Newacheck, "Childhood Asthma and Poverty: Differential Impacts and Utilization of Health Services," *Pediatrics*, Vol. 91, No. 1, 1993, pp. 56–61.

6. Lara, M., H. Morgenstern, N. Duan, and R. H. Brook, "Elevated Asthma Morbidity in Puerto Rican Children: A Review of Possible Risk and Prognostic Factors," *Western Journal of Medicine*, Vol. 170, No. 2, 1999, pp. 75–84.

7. Claudio, L., L. Tulton, J. Doucette, and P. J. Landrigan, "Socioeconomic Factors and Asthma Hospitalization Rates

in New York City,"*Journal of Asthma,* Vol. 36, No. 4, 1999, pp. 343–350.

8. Homa, D. M., D. M. Mannino, and M. Lara, "Asthma Mortality in U.S. Hispanics of Mexican, Puerto Rican, and Cuban Heritage, 1990–1995," *American Journal of Respiratory and Critical Care Medicine,* Vol. 161, No.2, Pt. 1, 2000, pp. 504–509.

9. Weiss, K. B., S. D. Sullivan, and C. S. Lyttle, "Trends in the Cost of Illness for Asthma in the United States, 1985–1994," *Journal of Allergy and Clinical Immunology,* Vol. 106, No. 3, 2000, pp. 493-500.

10. Weiss, K. B., P. J. Gergen, and T. A. Hodgson, "An Economic Evaluation of Asthma in the United States," *New England Journal of Medicine,* Vol. 326, No. 13, 1992, pp. 862–866.

11. PEW Environmental Health Commission, *Attack Asthma: Why America Needs a Public Health Defense System to Battle Environmental Threats,* 2000.

12. National Heart, Lung, and Blood Institute, National Asthma Education and Prevention Program, *Practical Guide for the Diagnosis and Management of Asthma: Based on the Expert Panel Report 2: Guidelines for the Diagnosis and Management of Asthma,* Bethesda, Md.: National Institutes of Health, U.S. Department of Health and Human Services. Pub. No. 97-4063, 1997.

13. Gern, J. E., R. J. Lemanske, and W. W. Busse, "Early Life Origins of Asthma," *Journal of Clinical Investigation,* Vol. 104, No. 7, 1999, pp. 837–843.

14. Institute of Medicine, *Clearing the Air: Asthma and Indoor Air Exposures,* Washington, D.C.: National Academy Press, 2000.

15. U.S. Census Bureau., *Poverty in the United States, 1999,* Washington, D.C., 2000, p. 8.

16. Halterman, J. S., C. A. Aligne, P. Auinger, J. T. McBride, and P. G. Szilagyi, "Inadequate Therapy for Asthma Among Children in the United States," *Pediatrics,* Vol. 105, No. 1, Pt. 3, 2000, pp. 272–276.

17. Laumann, J. M., and D. C. Bjornson, "Treatment of Medicaid Patients with Asthma: Comparison with Treatment Guidelines Using Disease-Based Drug Utilization Review Methodology," *Annals of Pharmacotherapy,* Vol. 32, No. 12, 1998, pp. 1290–1294.

18. Legorreta, A. P., J. Christian-Herman, R. D. O'Connor, M. M. Hasan, R. Evans, and K. M. Leung, "Compliance with National Asthma Management Guidelines and Specialty Care: A Health Maintenance Organization Experience," *Archives of Internal Medicine,* Vol. 158, No. 5, 1998, pp. 457–464.

19. Warman, K. L., E. J. Silver, M. P. McCourt, and R. E. K. Stein, "How Does Home Management of Asthma Exacerbations by Parents of Inner-City Children Differ from NHLBI (National Heart, Lung, and Blood Institute) Guideline Recommendations?" *Pediatrics,* Vol. 103, No. 2, 1999, pp. 422–427.

20. Lewis, M. A., G. Rachelefsky, C. E. Lewis, B. Leake, and W. Richards, "The Termination of a Randomized Clinical Trial for Poor Hispanic Children," *Archives of Pediatrics and Adolescent Medicine,* Vol. 148, No. 4, 1994, pp. 364–367.

21. Finkelstein, J. A., R. W. Brown, L. C. Schneider, et al., "Quality of Care for Preschool Children with Asthma: The Role of Social Factors and Practice Setting," *Pediatrics,* Vol. 95, No. 3, 1995, pp. 389–394.

22. Homer, C. J., P. Szilagyi, L. Rodewald, et al., "Does Quality of Care Affect Rates of Hospitalization for Childhood Asthma?" *Pediatrics,* Vol. 98, No. 1, 1996, pp. 18–23.

23. Crain, E. F., C. Kercsmar, K. B. Weiss, H. Mitchell, and H. Lynn, "Reported Difficulties in Access to Quality Care for Children with Asthma in the Inner City," *Archives of Pediatrics and Adolescent Medicine,* Vol. 152, No. 4, 1998, pp. 333–339.

24. Kattan, M., H. Mitchell, P. Eggleston, et al., "Characteristics of Inner-City Children with Asthma: The National Cooperative Inner-City Asthma Study," *Pediatric Pulmonology,* Vol. 24, No. 4, 1997, pp. 253–262.

25. Lara, M., F. Allen, and L. Lange, "Physician Perceptions of Barriers to Care for Inner-City Latino Children with Asthma," *Journal of Health Care for the Poor and Underserved,* Vol. 10, No. 1, 1999, pp. 27–44.

26. Eggleston, P. A., F. J. Malveaux, A. M. Butz, et al., "Medications Used by Children with Asthma Living in the Inner City," *Pediatrics,* Vol. 101, No. 3, 1998, pp. 349–354.

27. Evans, D., R. Mellins, K. Lobach, et al., "Improving Care for Minority Children with Asthma: Professional Education in Public Health Clinics," *Pediatrics,* Vol. 99, No. 2, 1997, pp. 157–164.

28. Greineder, D. K., K. C. Loane, and P. Parks, "A Randomized Controlled Trial of a Pediatric Asthma Outreach Program," *Journal of Allergy and Clinical Immunology,* Vol. 103, No. 3, 1999, pp. 436–440.

29. Evans, R., P. J. Gergen, H. Mitchell, et al., "A Randomized Clinical Trial to Reduce Asthma Morbidity Among Inner-City Children: Results of the National Cooperative Inner-City Asthma Study," *Journal of Pediatrics,* Vol. 135, No. 3, 1999, pp. 332–338.

30. Sullivan, S. D., and K. B. Weiss, "Health Economics of Asthma and Rhinitis. II. Assessing the Value of Interventions," *Journal of Allergy and Clinical Immunology,* Vol. 107, 2001, pp. 203–210.

31. Environmental Protection Agency, Office of Air and Radiation, Office of Radiation and Indoor Air, Indoor Environment Division (6609J), *Internal Air Quality Tools for Schools: Managing Asthma in the School Environment,* Research Triangle Park, N.C., EPA No. 402-K-00-0003, May 2000.

32. U.S. Department of Health and Human Services, *Healthy People 2010,* Washington, D.C.

33. American Lung Association and American Thoracic Society, Government Relations Office, *Action on Asthma,* 2000.

34. Asthma and Allergy Foundation of America, *Costs of Asthma in America, 2000* (www.aafa.org/highcosts/index.html).

35. Allergy and Asthma Network/Mothers of Asthmatics, Inc., "Asthma Awareness Day, Capitol Hill 2000 Proves Asthma Is Serious," 2000 (www.aanma.org).

36. American Academy of Allergy, Asthma, and Immunology Taskforce, *Pediatric Asthma: Promoting Best Practice: Guide for Managing Asthma in Children,* 1999.

37. NCQA, "Asthma Measurement Advisory Panel," 2000 (www.ncqa.org/Pages/Programs/HEDIS/index.htm).

38. Jones, J., and D. Hunter, "Consensus Methods for Medical and Health Services Research," *BMJ* (Clinical Research Ed.), Vol. 311, No. 7001, 1995, pp. 376–380.

39. Lara, M., and C. Goodman, *National Priorities for the Assessment of Clinical Conditions and Medical Technologies: Report of a Pilot Study,* Washington, D.C.: National Academy Press, Institute of Medicine Publication IOM-89-14, 1990.

40. Andersen, R. M. "Revisiting the Behavioral Model and Access to Medical Care: Does It Matter?" *Journal of Health and Social Behavior,* Vol. 36, No. 1, 1995, pp. 1–10.

41. Clark, N. M., "Management of Asthma by Parents and Children," in H. Kotses and A. Harver, eds., *Self-Management of Asthma,* New York: Marcel Dekker, Inc., 1998, pp. 271–291.

42. Comino, E. J., C. A. Mitchell, A. Bauman, et al., "Asthma Management in Eastern Australia, 1990 and 1993," *Medical Journal of Australia,* Vol. 164, No. 7, 1996, pp. 403–406.

43. National Heart, Lung, and Blood Institute, National Asthma Education and Prevention Program, School Asthma Education Subcommittee, "How Asthma Friendly Is Your School?" *Journal of School Health,* Vol. 68, No. 4, 1998, pp. 167–168.

44. Platts-Mills, T. A., D. Vervloet, W. R. Thomas, R. C. Aalberse, and M. D. Chapman, "Indoor Allergens and Asthma: Report of the Third International Workshop," *Journal of Allergy and Clinical Immunology,* Vol. 100, No. 6, Pt. 1, 1997, pp. S2–24.

45. Newacheck, P. W., and B. Starfield, "Morbidity and Use of Ambulatory Care Services Among Poor and Nonpoor Children," *American Journal of Public Health,* Vol. 78, No. 8, 1988, pp. 927–933.

46. U.S. Census Bureau, *Current Population Coverage, Health Insurance Coverage,* Washington, D.C., 2000.

47. Flores, G., M. Abreu, M. A. Olivar, and B. Kastner, "Access Barriers to Health Care for Latino Children," *Archives of Pediatrics and Adolescent Medicine,* Vol. 152, No. 11, 1998, pp. 1119–1125.

48. Kibbe, D. C., A. D. Kaluzny, and C. P. McLaughlin, "Integrating Guidelines with Continuous Quality Improvement: Doing the Right Thing the Right Way to Achieve the Right Goals," *Joint Commission Journal on Quality Improvement,* Vol. 20, No. 4, 1994, pp. 181–191.

49. Kaluzny, A. D., T. R. Konrad, and C. P. McLaughlin, "Organizational Strategies for Implementing Clinical Guidelines [see comments]," *Joint Commission Journal on Quality Improvement,* Vol. 21, No. 7, 1995, pp. 347–351.

50. Bero, L. A., R. Grilli, J. M Grimshaw, E. Harvey, A. D. Oxman, and M. A. Thomson (The Cochrane Effective Practice and Organization of Care Review Group), "Closing the Gap Between Research and Practice: An Overview of Systematic Reviews of Interventions to Promote the Implementation of Research Findings," *BMJ* (Clinical Research Ed.), Vol. 317, No. 7156, 1998, pp. 465–468.

51. Clark, N. M., D. Evans, B. J. Zimmerman, M. J. Levison, and R. B. Mellins, "Patient and Family Management of Asthma: Theory-Based Techniques for the Clinician," *Journal of Asthma,* Vol. 31, No. 6, 1994, pp. 427–435.

52. Conboy, K., "Self-Management Skills for Cooperative Care in Asthma," *Journal of Pediatrics,* Vol. 115, No. 5, Pt. 2, 1989, pp. 863–866.

53. Wolf, F. M., C. M. Grum, and N. M. Clark, "Educational Interventions for Children with Asthma," *Cochrane Electronic Library,* 2000.

54. Greineder, D. K., K. C. Loane, and P. Parks, "Reduction in Resource Utilization by an Asthma Outreach Program," *Archives of Pediatrics and Adolescent Medicine,* Vol. 149, No. 4, 1995, pp. 415–420.

55. Sullivan, S., A. Elixhauser, A. S. Buist, B. R. Luce, J. Eisenberg, and K. B. Weiss, "National Asthma Education and Prevention Program Working Group Report on the Cost Effectiveness of Asthma Care," *American Journal of Respiratory and Critical Care Medicine,* Vol. 154, No. 3, Pt. 2, 1996, pp. S84–S95.

56. Kelso, T. M., N. Abou-shala, G. M. Heilker, et al., "Comprehensive Long-Term Management Program for Asthma: Effect on Outcomes in Adult African Americans," *American Journal of Medical Science,* Vol. 311, No. 6, 1996, pp. 272–280.

57. Munroe, W. P., K. Kunz, et al., "Economic Evaluation of Pharmacist Involvement in Disease Management in a Community Pharmacy Setting," *Clinical Therapist,* Vol. 19, No. 1, 1997, pp. 113–123.

58. Moyer, P., "Low Hanging Fruit: Asthma Is Seen As Easy Pickings in the Disease Management Orchard. So Is Asthma Therapy by Pharmacists a Good Way to Approach Cognitive Services?" *Managed Healthcare,* September 1995, pp. S11–S12, 48.

59. Bodenheimer, T., "Disease Management—Promises and Pitfalls," *New England Journal of Medicine,* Vol. 340, No. 15, 1999, pp. 1202–1205.

60. Epstein, R. S., and L .M. Sherwood, "From Outcomes Research to Disease Management: A Guide for the Perplexed," *Annals of Internal Medicine,* Vol. 124, No. 9, 1996, pp. 832–837.

61. Pauley, T. R., M. J. Magee, and J. D. Cury, "Pharmacist-Managed Physician Directed Asthma Management Program Reduces Emergency Department Visits," *American Pharmacotherapy,* Vol. 29, 1995, pp. 5–9.

62. Rupp, M. T., D. J. McCallian, and K. K. Sheth, "Developing and Marketing a Community Pharmacy-based Asthma Management Program," *Journal of the American Pharmaceutical Association*, Vol. NS37, 1997, pp. 694–699.

63. Kelly, C. S., A. L. Morrow, J. Shults, N. Nakas, G. L. Strope, and R. D. Adelman, "Outcomes Evaluation of a Comprehensive Intervention Program for Asthmatic Children Enrolled in Medicaid," *Pediatrics*, Vol. 105, No. 5, 2000, pp. 1029–1035.

64. Kattan, M., E. F. Crain, and H. Mitchell, "Frequent Users vs. Non-Users of the Emergency Department Among Inner-City Children with Asthma," *American Journal of Respiratory and Critical Care Medicine*, Vol. 155, No. 4, 1997, p. A283.

65. *The Kaiser Commission on Medicaid and the Uninsured, Uninsured in America*, The Henry J. Kaiser Family Foundation, 2000.

66. Rosenbaum, S., A. Markus, and D. Roby, *An Analysis of Implementation Issues Relating to SCHIP Cost-Sharing Provisions for Certain Targeted Low Income Children*, Prepared for the Health Care Financing Administration and the Health Resources and Services Administration Under Contract No. 98-OA-140506, 1999.

67. Newacheck, P. W., J. J. Stoddard, D. C. Hughes, and M. Pearl, "Health Insurance and Access to Primary Care for Children," *New England Journal of Medicine*, Vol. 338, No. 8, 1998, pp. 513–519.

68. Sumner, B., and N. Lurie, "Financial Payment Systems and Asthma Care," *Medical Care*, Vol. 31, No. 3, Suppl., 1993, pp. MS74–MS81.

69. Ellis, E. R., and V. K. Smith, *Medicaid Enrollment in 21 States, June 1997 to June 1999*, Lansing, Michigan: Health Management Associates, 1-80, 2000.

70. Brown, E., R. Wyn, H. Yu, A. Valenzuela, and L. Dong, "Access to Health Insurance and Health Care for Children in Immigrant Families," in D. J. Hernandez, ed., *Children of Immigrants:*

Health, Adjustment, and Public Assistance, Washington, D.C.: National Academy Press, 1998, pp. 126–132.

71. Rosenbaum, S., K. Johnson, C. Sonosky, A. Markus, and C. DeGraw, "The Children's Hour: The State Children's Health Insurance Program," *Health Affairs,* Vol. 17, No. 1, 1998, pp. 75–89.

72. Liptak, G. S., C. M. Burns, P. W. Davidson, and E. R. McAnarney, "Effects of Providing Comprehensive Ambulatory Services to Children with Chronic Conditions," *Archives of Pediatrics and Adolescent Medicine,* Vol. 152, No. 10, 1998, pp. 1003–1008.

73. Schauffler, H. H., and T. Rodriguez, "Exercising Purchasing Power for Preventive Care," *Health Affairs,* Vol. 15, No. 1, 1996, pp. 73–85.

74. Newacheck, P. W., and N. Halfon, "Prevalence, Impact, and Trends in Childhood Disability Due to Asthma," *Archives of Pediatrics and Adolescent Medicine,* Vol. 154, No. 3, 2000, pp. 287–293.

75. Fillmore, E. J., N. Jones, and J. M. Blankson, "Achieving Treatment Goals for Schoolchildren with Asthma," *Archives of Disease in Childhood,* Vol. 77, No. 5, 1997, pp. 420–422.

76. Thies, K. M., "Identifying the Educational Implications of Chronic Illness in School Children," *Journal of School Health,* Vol. 69, No. 10, 1999, pp. 392–397.

77. Weiss, K. B., and S. D. Sullivan, "The Economic Costs of Asthma: A Review and Conceptual Model," *Pharmacoeconomics,* Vol. 4, No. 1, 1993, pp. 14–30.

78. Pettersson, E., A. Gardulf, G. Nordstrom, C. Svanberg-Johnsson, and G. Bylin, "Evaluation of a Nurse-Run Asthma School," *International Journal of Nursing Studies,* Vol. 36, No. 2, 1999, pp. 145–151.

79. Meurer, J. R., S. McKenzie, E. Mischler, S. Subichin, M. Malloy, and V. George, "The Awesome Asthma School Days Program: Educating Children, Inspiring a Community," *Journal of School Health,* Vol. 69, No. 2, 1999, pp. 63–68.

80. Lurie, N., M. J. Straub, N. Goodman, and E. J. Bauer, "Incorporating Asthma Education into a Traditional School Curriculum," *American Journal of Public Health*, Vol. 88, No. 5, 1998, pp. 822–823.

81. Christiansen, S. C., S. B. Martin, N. C. Schleicher, J. A. Koziol, K. P. Mathews, and B. L. Zuraw, "Evaluation of a School-based Asthma Education Program for Inner-City Children," *Journal of Allergy and Clinical Immunology*, Vol. 100, No. 5, 1997, pp. 613–617.

82. McEwen, M., P. Johnson, J. Neatherlin, M. W. Millard, and G. Lawrence, "School-based Management of Chronic Asthma Among Inner-City African-American Schoolchildren in Dallas, Texas," *Journal of School Health*, Vol. 68, No. 5, 1998, pp. 196–201.

83. State of Maryland, *Code of Maryland Regulations 13A.05.05.05 School Health Service Standards*, Annapolis, Md., 2000.

84. U.S. Supreme Court, *Cedar Rapids Community School District v. Garret F.*, No. 96-1793, 2000.

85. Centers for Disease Control, "Forecasted State-Specific Estimates of Self-Reported Asthma Prevalence—United States, 1998," *MMWR*, Vol. 47, No. 47, 1998, pp. 1022–1025.

86. Grant, E. N., J. N. Moy, K. Turner-Roan, S. R. Daugherty, and K. B. Weiss (Chicago Asthma Surveillance Initiative Project Team), "Asthma Care Practices, Perceptions, and Beliefs of Chicago-Area Primary-Care Physicians," *Chest*, Vol. 116, No. 4, Suppl. 1, 1999, pp. 145S–154S.

87. Comino, E. J., A. Bauman, C. A. Mitchell, et al., "The Australian National Asthma Campaign: Effects of Public Education Activities Based on Mass Media," *American Journal of Preventive Medicine*, Vol. 13, No. 4, 1997, pp. 251–256.

88. McCaul, K. A., M. A Wakefield,. D. M. Roder, et al., "Trends in Hospital Readmission for Asthma: Has the Australian National Asthma Campaign Had an Effect?" *Medical Journal of Australia*, Vol. 172, No. 2, 2000, pp. 62–66.

89. Centers for Disease Control, "Asthma Surveillance Programs in Public Health Departments—United States," *MMWR,* Vol. 45, No. 37, 1996, pp. 802–804.

90. Custovic, A., A. Simpson, M. D. Chapman, and A. Woodcock, "Allergen Avoidance in the Treatment of Asthma and Atopic Disorders," *Thorax,* Vol. 53, No. 1, 1998, pp. 63–72.

91. Gergen, P. J., J. A. Fowler, K. R. Maurer, W. W. Davis, and M. D. Overpeck, "The Burden of Environmental Tobacco Smoke Exposure on the Respiratory Health of Children 2 Months Through 5 Years of Age in the United States: Third National Health and Nutrition Examination Survey, 1988 to 1994," *Pediatrics,* Vol. 101, No. 2, 1998, p. E8.

92. Hide, D. W., S. Matthews, S. Tariq,and S. H. Arshad, "Allergen Avoidance in Infancy and Allergy at 4 Years of Age," *Allergy,* Vol. 51, No. 2, 1996, pp. 89–93.

93. Platts-Mills, T. A., and M. C. Carter, "Asthma and Indoor Exposure to Allergens," *New England Journal of Medicine,* Vol. 336, No. 19, 1997, pp. 1382–1384.

94. Litonjua, A. A., V. J. Carey, S. T. Weiss, and D. R. Gold, "Race, Socioeconomic Factors, and Area of Residence Are Associated with Asthma Prevalence," *Pediatric Pulmonology,* Vol. 28, No. 6, 1999, pp. 394–401.

95. Miller, J. E., "The Effects of Race/Ethnicity and Income on Early Childhood Asthma Prevalence and Health Care Use," *American Journal of Public Health,* Vol. 90, No. 3, 2000, pp. 428–430.

Made in the USA
Coppell, TX
28 September 2021

63135726R10073